"*Your Body Never Meant You Any Harm* is a profoundly healing book. It guides readers to transform their sometimes painful and conflicted relationship with their bodies through the power of self-compassion and forgiveness. With warmth, clarity, and wisdom, it shows that the body is not the enemy—it's a loyal ally that has been trying to protect us all along. In doing so, it offers a path to genuine wholeness and freedom."

—Kristin Neff, PhD, author of *Self-Compassion* and *Fierce Self-Compassion*

"This is a book about coming home. Coming home to yourself and coming home to the wisdom deep within your flesh. In a world full of rupture, the pages within provide essential guidance to mend the mind and body split while providing insightful care on the path to healing and self-love."

—Tias Little, MA, author of *Yoga of the Subtle Body*

"This book is guaranteed to change how you relate to your body. It is intuitive and informed, wise and compassionate—the culmination of Dr. Biasetti's years of commitment to understanding the complicated relationship we have with our bodies. She gently guides the reader through ten stages on the path to body forgiveness. Every word is carefully chosen to help us remember the compassionate relationship we had with our bodies when we were born. Get ready to be touched, moved, and uplifted by what you read."

—Christopher Germer, PhD, lecturer at Harvard Medical School and author of *Self-Compassion for Shame*

"This book is a compassionate companion for any woman learning to come home to herself. Dr. Saffi Biasetti writes with the warmth of a wise teacher and the precision of someone who has both lived and lovingly facilitated the process of coming home to your body. Rooted in self-compassion research and somatic practice, this book offers gentle guidance for anyone ready to be led back home to their body."

—Ailey Jolie, MCP, MA, somatic psychologist

"This book outlines a lovely path to developing a relationship with your body and heal from societal messages as well as personal experiences and patterns of disconnection. Designed particularly for women who struggle with body connection and/or disordered eating, Dr. Saffi Biasetti draws on her personal journey and her professional expertise, guiding the reader with compassionate encouragement to explore the promise of an embodied life."

—Cynthia Price, PhD, MA, LMT,
director of the Center for Mindful Body Awareness

"This book gets under the skin of the relationship we all have with our bodies. It is a deep dive into the subtleties of our amazing ability to communicate through our cells. It is full of hope as it guides us through the possibilities of a forgiving and compassionate relationship with ourselves. Dr. Saffi Biasetti takes our hand in hers on the healing path to a more rich, joyful, and profound life. I highly recommend this book as a reminder of the possibility of living in love and at peace with your precious, unique body."

—Galia Tyano Ronen, LCP, coeditor and coauthor of
Grounding Psychotherapy in Self-Compassion

"In *Your Body Never Meant You Any Harm*, Dr. Saffi Biasetti serves as a steady and insightful guide through terrain that is both intimate and universal. With depth and compassion, she offers a thoughtfully constructed map for reconnecting with the body as a source of insight rather than conflict. Through poignant stories and gently unfolding practices, abstract ideals such as self-compassion and forgiveness become embodied, lived realities. This book restores the body to its rightful place—not as an adversary to be managed, but as a loving companion, sacred teacher, and enduring source of healing."

—Patty Hlava, PhD, professor and lead core faculty
of the PhD and MATP programs at Sofia University

"There is real relief in these pages—the sense of being understood rather than corrected. Dr. Saffi Biasetti offers a steady, compassionate invitation back into a relationship with the body, making it feel natural to remember that it was never the problem to begin with."

—Stefanie Michele, occupational therapist,
Somatic Experiencing Practitioner,
and certified intuitive eating counselor

YOUR BODY NEVER MEANT YOU ANY HARM

A Somatic Guide to Forgiving and Healing
Your Relationship with Your Body

ANN SAFFI BIASETTI, PHD, LCSW

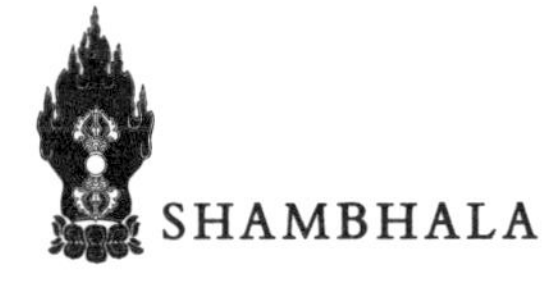

Shambhala Publications, Inc.
2129 13th Street
Boulder, Colorado 80302
www.shambhala.com

Cover art: Coffee Cafe Lover / Adobe Stock
Cover design: Daniel Urban-Brown
Interior design: Laura Shaw Design

9 8 7 6 5 4 3 2 1

First Edition
Printed in the United States of America

Shambhala Publications makes every effort to print on acid-free,
recycled paper. Shambhala Publications is distributed worldwide by
Penguin Random House, Inc., and its subsidiaries.

Library of Congress Cataloging-in-Publication Data
ISBN 978-1-64547-441-8
LC record available at https://lccn.loc.gov/2025049248.

The authorized representative in the EU for product safety and
compliance is eucomply OÜ, Pärnu mnt 139b-14, 11317 Tallinn, Estonia,
hello@eucompliancepartner.com.

I dedicate this book to my daughter Olivia, who inspires me daily with her strength, wisdom, and ability to show up in the world just as she is. I hope that together we have learned to break the intergenerational cycle of disembodiment. May you continue to live freely and fully embodied.

———————

To my mom, who passed away during the writing of this book. I love you and know you did your best to be free. May you now be free from pain and suffering.

———————

To the brave women who volunteered to participate in the Body Forgiveness Project. Many wondered whether they were ready to be a part of it. I hope this book demonstrates that they were exactly where they needed to be.

———————

To my clients and the many women who have participated in my Befriending Your Body Program and retreats. You inspire me to keep doing what I do.

———————

Lastly, I express immense gratitude to my spiritual practice and the many teachers who have influenced my journey of body forgiveness and embodiment. My body and I thank you.

and i said to my body. softly. "i want to be your friend." it took a long breath. and replied "i have been waiting my whole life for this."

—Nayyirah Waheed

CONTENTS

YOUR BODY NEVER MEANT YOU ANY HARM

INTRODUCTION

Thank you for having the courage to pick up this book. I know it is not easy to read a book titled *Your Body Never Meant You Any Harm*, and I imagine you want to do so because these words resonate with you in some way. They carry different meanings for everyone. For some, these words bring up feelings of sadness and grief, prompting tears; for others, they provoke anger, rage, and regret. Some may feel curiosity, relief, and awe, while others experience joy, a sense of spirit, gratitude, and a deeper connection.

You may feel these words resonating deep within your body, as words don't just land in our minds but also land in our bodies. You will come to understand and feel this throughout this book. With these words, you may notice something moving inside you or being touched in a certain way. Perhaps you experience warmth or an intense sensation, like muscles tensing or tightening. Or you might find tears forming and experience a tenderness, relief, and sense of letting go in your body. You may notice a rush of thoughts and memories flooding your mind, or you might find a sense of internal peace and gratitude emerging.

However the title landed in you, there is a reason you chose this book. Each of us has a unique relationship with our body and a story that has a long history, perhaps longer than you realize. You don't need to understand this reason or the story right now—helping you discover those things is the focus of part one of this book. For now, whatever you notice is valuable information from your body about this moment. This will also shift, change, and—we hope—evolve into something new, as long as a part of you is open and curious to learn more.

Your Body Never Meant You Any Harm is a psychospiritual, somatic guide that helps you reconnect with one of the most important relationships in your life: the one that you have with your body. How did we go from being born as fully embodied, deeply connected, sensing and feeling individuals to feeling disconnected from our bodies or even at war with them? How did we come to feel shame, hatred, disgust, fear, disappointment, and betrayal toward our bodies? What caused the disruption and severance that has led so many of us to feel disconnected, even though separation is not our natural state? And how might we find our way back into a relationship with our bodies based on intimacy, kindness, gentleness, balance, intuition, and connection?

I don't expect you to have all the answers, or any, to these questions; all of us need guidance and support to help us navigate our way back. If you do have some answers, I'm thrilled that you've discovered them, and this book can help you find even more. And if you find yourself without answers, as most women do, this book is especially for you. The embodied practices and reflections in this book offer you a way to answer these questions and more. They will help you understand that the true nature of your body is forgiving, compassionate, and spiritual—it always has been. You will learn what led you away from your body and what can bring you back.

However, if you are like most women, you may feel lost, confused, and uncertain about what it even means to develop a relationship with your body and whether you are capable of doing so. You might blame yourself, believing that you have done something wrong, that you are too much or not enough. Many women find themselves in a cycle of constant blame toward their bodies, feeling as if their bodies are the reason they experience certain emotions or face problems in their lives and relationships. Please note that it's normal to feel this way right now, and you are not alone.

Embodiment is the process of developing an intimate relationship with your body. I have wanted to write a book on this topic for a very long time because I have lived this journey myself; and for more than three decades as a somatic psychotherapist, transpersonal psychologist, and yoga therapist, I have helped thousands of women find their way back into relationship with their bodies after living disconnected for so long. Over the years I developed a form of somatic psychotherapy called embodied self-compassion. Embodied self-compassion encompasses everything you will learn in this book: somatic skills grounded in interoceptive awareness, the transformative power of compassion to foster safety and security within your body, and the journey toward reestablishing a relationship with your body, which will become your most protective healer over time.

The lack of relationship you have with your body—and the sense of disconnection and separation you have from it—is known as disembodiment. This feeling, which you will learn more about in chapter 1, isn't something you created or desired. Rather, it is a learned response influenced by cultural norms, especially for women, and reinforced for generations. By picking up this book you are already engaging in a radical countercultural act: seeking to understand your body, and the bodies of the women who came before you, in a new way.

What Is Body Forgiveness?

While it might seem strange to think of your body as something you can develop a relationship with, that is precisely what body forgiveness entails. Whether you realize it or not, there was a time when you had a close connection with your body. Even if you can't remember it, you were born with an intimate bond to your physical self. You came into the world as an embodied being—fully connected, sensing, feeling, knowing, and present—completely integrated and in harmony with your body. Body forgiveness is an iterative process for reconnecting and building that relationship. By moving through the stages in order and engaging in the exercises and reflections, you will gradually reengage with your body and release old stories.

The term *forgiveness*, as I am using it, carries a different meaning than what you may be accustomed to. Typically, forgiveness implies that we must let go of something that has wronged or hurt us. You and your body have not done anything wrong. Neither you nor your body has caused any offense. Many factors contributed to the rupture of your relationship with your body, and none of them originated with you. Part one of this book will help you clarify and understand how your beliefs about your body developed through the messages you absorbed from the world around you and from your personal experiences. The disconnection, separation, and detachment you may have experienced often stem from ingrained beliefs about your body that were never truly yours. These beliefs have pulled you away from what should have been an intimate and natural relationship with your body.

I coined the term *body forgiveness* after conducting my first qualitative research study on the role of self-compassion and embodiment in women recovering from eating disorders. In this study many participants emphasized the significance of forgiveness, which allowed self-compassion to flourish. This research eventually led to my first book, *Befriending Your Body: A Self-Compassionate Approach to Freeing Yourself from Disordered Eating*. From this work I developed a somatic recovery program called The Befriending Your Body Program. It was in the middle of guiding my first program that I identified and recognized the importance of body forgiveness, and I longed to know more.

During that first program, I guided the group through a meditation on forgiveness. In the subsequent discussion and feedback session, many people shared that they struggled to forgive themselves for past mistakes and behaviors and felt a sense of confusion toward their bodies. This struggle left them feeling blocked and stuck.

Practicing forgiveness toward our bodies can feel impossible when we are confronted with intense emotions like anger, resentment, disgust, loathing, and betrayal. I could sense the heaviness among the group as they came up against barriers I was all too familiar with from my own past. It's a block that develops over years of feeling disembodied, as if your mind and body are separate entities, and it leaves you feeling like you no longer recognize your own body. That day the group felt blocked, and the concept of forgiveness seemed forced and filled with shame. Their minds were consumed by all the wrongs they believed they had committed against their bodies. They were focused on the past rather than the present moment, trying to force forgiveness from their minds, willing it to be the truth.

In that moment, I said simply what came to mind, "I know this is hard, but please understand, your body never meant you any harm." Yes, I used the exact words that may have enticed you to pick up this book.

After I said those words, something shifted. I didn't know exactly what had changed, only that the impact was profound. I could see, feel, and sense it in my participants and their bodies. Forgiveness from the body does just that. It creates an internal shift. Unlike forgiving from our minds, body forgiveness produces an immense physical release and brings relief to your body and your mind. The process laid out in this book will be the groundwork for guiding you to experiencing body forgiveness yourself in chapter 7.

That evening marked a significant shift for my students. I, too, was inspired and wanted to understand more about what had caused such a shift. As a qualitative researcher, I am interested in the lived experience of people, not just numbers. After spending a few more years delivering my program and watching people shift from shame, blame, and regret into compassion for themselves and their bodies, I decided to embark on another qualitative research study.

In 2023 I conducted an independent qualitative research study titled The Body Forgiveness Project. Twenty self-identified females volunteered to participate. While I did not set out to interview only women, that is who came forward to join the study. As I spent time with the study participants, they increasingly expressed the need for women to develop a new understanding of and relationship with their bodies. They yearned for compassion, community, and connection rather than competition and comparison. Moreover, they emphasized the need for a safe space where women could learn about and explore the path of body forgiveness and embodiment.

As most women can attest, this journey has been uniquely challenging. As a result, I decided to focus this book on anyone assigned female at birth or who identifies as female—I refer to these groups as "women" throughout the book. That said, the insights and guidance in this book are valuable for anyone. I strongly encourage those who identify as male or who were assigned male at birth to read this book to gain a deeper understanding, connect with, and honor the women in their lives who are striving for reembodiment. These men may also find similarities or parallels to their own lived experience.

I began each interview in the study by asking my participants to reflect on the words that seemed to hold the magic: "Your body never meant you any harm." I invited them to notice their internal, embodied response to the words. Their responses are woven throughout the pages of this book, bringing the journey of embodiment to life. I learned a great deal from their stories and their lived experiences, which revealed the intense challenges of moving from separation and disembodiment to compassion, forgiveness, and embodiment. Because of their willingness to be vulnerable and share deeply, I was able to identify the ten stages of body forgiveness. I am deeply grateful to them and consider them cocreators of this work—you will find quotes from them throughout the book.

The journey of body forgiveness is not a linear path but an ongoing, iterative process that unfolds in stages. Each part of this book builds upon the previous, inviting you to move through the material in order—layer by layer—so that each new insight and practice can be integrated fully before moving forward. Please feel free to take your time with each chapter, revisiting any sections along the way as you need. As one study participant shared, "It's not about doing or having done something wrong. You have to think about forgiveness differently." With this in mind, the book is designed to gently guide you through understanding, embodying, and ultimately embracing a new relationship with your body.

Part One: Understanding lays the foundation by offering a new perspective on your relationship with your body. You will explore the roots of disembodiment, learn what embodiment really means, and develop an understanding of your sensory experiences and the internal narrative of your body. We will explore, with gentleness and curiosity, the internal and external influences that have shaped your relationship with your body.

Part Two: Embodying introduces essential practical actions you can take to support your journey to embodiment. This section emphasizes the importance of self-compassion as the necessary first step before taking you through practices to help you meet difficult emotions such as grief, regret, and shame with kindness and presence—transforming them from sources of pain into opportunities for healing. Through these steps you will begin to experience the process of forgiveness as something that is embodied rather than just understood intellectually.

Part Three: Embracing focuses on what is necessary to sustain and nurture an embodied life. Here you will explore what it means to remain present and connected to your body, even during diffi-cult times. You will learn how to embrace the impermanence of bodily sensations, thoughts, and feelings, as well as how to cultivate equanimity, presence, and a sense of community—all to support a lifelong practice of returning to your body with compassion and acceptance.

Rediscovering My Connection to My Body

I rediscovered my connection to my body many years ago after struggling with body disconnection for decades. As a teenager, after going through several traumatic events (the type of events I call "exceptional experiences"), I had little understanding of how these experiences had affected my body. The only awareness I had was of how they impacted my mind. This is not uncommon, as we are often taught to move away from the innate internal knowledge we are born with and instead rely on our thoughts to make sense of our experiences. But our bodies will continue to communicate with us until we finally listen.

I was a shy and sensitive child, easily affected by my surroundings. My body was also quite sensitive in responding to the environment around me. I coped with these exceptional experiences by becoming quiet and avoiding attention, particularly in public and at school. Despite feeling small inside, this didn't stop my classmates from noticing my smallness—both in my voice and my physique—and they made it clear that they saw both as problems or as something wrong. My home life was filled with sadness and anxiety, which manifested in my body as stomachaches, constipation, a racing heart, and nightmares. I carried a deep sadness but tried to cope with it by being irritable and angry, as that felt safer than the vulnerability of sadness and fear. I desperately hoped someone at home would recognize what I was experiencing and acknowledge the issues within the family. They didn't.

By the time I turned fifteen, that sadness and fear filled my body with an overwhelming energy, what I would later refer to as a state of *overdrive*. (I discuss this idea in chapter 4.) At the time, I interpreted this state as anxiety and stress. I was moving through life with a sense of urgency and a drive for survival, and I was impelled by perfectionism, which left me constantly feeling off-center and ungrounded. Slowing down was beyond challenging for me and felt like a nonnegotiable.

When I was sixteen my father tragically passed away after years of battling alcoholism, and my body collapsed into a state I can only describe as *underdrive*. (I discuss this idea in chapter 4 too.) I was unaccustomed to this feeling. What was this darkness and heaviness that enveloped me? My mind struggled to comprehend it. I felt an increasing sense of fear as the internal heaviness grew, along with the anxiety that my body, on the cusp of young adulthood, was going to be the next thing to change in my life. I felt I could not survive another change.

Simultaneously I was inundated by the messages of diet culture that had taken the 1980s by storm. In an unconscious effort to achieve some internal balance and find homeostasis for my body, I began restricting my food intake. Driven by fear of my changing body, I felt increasing distress. I wanted to disappear while still being seen, held, and loved at the same time. Food became my way of coping with a life and world that felt unsafe and threatening to my body.

My body cried out for internal stability and regulation. It was also yearning for gentleness and compassionate understanding, but I didn't know where to find that, having already been separated from myself. I often wonder what might have been different during those years if someone had told me, "My dear, you have endured so much. Your body and mind are just tired. You need to rest. You need to cry. You need a break. Your body is signaling that it needs to slow down and be nurtured for a while." This is what I have since learned to do whenever my body becomes overwhelmed by life. However, I didn't know this at the time, and no one shared that message with me.

I struggled for many years until I was met with kindness. That kindness came in the form of compassion from those around me, and eventually I learned to extend that compassion to myself. At the time, I didn't fully understand what this kindness meant. I only realized its impact by the way my body responded when someone truly saw and understood my pain. Slowly, I noticed that when I acknowledged and named my pain, something would also shift inside me.

In chapter 5 you will read about the transformative power of self-compassion and its effect on both your body and mind. I felt the effects of self-compassion as a release and a softening within myself. My fear would diminish, even if just for a moment, allowing me to properly nourish my body, which had been longing for care. Things were shifting: For now, my body and I were healing.

Many years later, at twenty-seven, I was trying to get pregnant. I had always wanted to be a mom, but my body was signaling that something wasn't right. Neither I nor my doctors understood what was wrong. I embarked on a journey of fertility treatments and, after three years, I became pregnant with twin boys. I was thrilled, but my body wasn't.

After their birth I was riding the new mother high, but my body was unable to maintain balance. The only way it seemed to communicate was through my breast milk. I was overproducing, which made it difficult to nurse my babies. I was told that this was a result of a twin birth and instructed to pump multiple times a day. As I juggled these demands, I began to lose my new mother high and my body became depleted and exhausted. I continued to push through, having been conditioned since childhood—perhaps even before that—to ignore my body's signals for rest and switch into the only survival mode I knew: overdrive.

Four months after giving birth, I could no longer ignore the signals my body was sending me. My body felt as if it were on fire, and I was in constant discomfort. I couldn't sleep, and despite eating large amounts of food, I was losing weight. Something was wrong. This wasn't the typical overdrive energy I was used to. I sought medical attention but was repeatedly told that my symptoms were simply due to anxiety and stress. While I wanted to trust the professionals, I was confused. The messages from my body were so intense that I was left either mistrusting my doctors or mistrusting my body.

I had no idea that I was experiencing numerous messages and screams from my body's internal awareness. Like many people, I often turned to my mind to decipher what I was feeling. Since I had a history of anxiety and panic attacks, I initially accepted the doctor's explanation. But what troubled me was how different this feeling was from the fear and panic I had experienced before. The feeling in my body didn't align with the explanation of stress that I was receiving from others. I often walked away feeling frustrated, invisible, and unheard. Nevertheless, I was complacent and compliant and ignored what I truly needed. I yearned to be acknowledged and understood, but I was searching in the wrong places.

My body was sending powerful messages, but I didn't know how to interpret them. I sensed that something was wrong and that it was profoundly affecting my feelings, thoughts, and actions. My heart raced as if it were going a mile a minute, and at thirty years old I feared I was having a heart attack. I struggled to walk up a flight of stairs without needing to sit down halfway to catch my breath. Despite these clear physical symptoms, my mind sided with the doctors and insisted that I was imagining it: "You're fine," "It's just stress," or "You're just tired." I was constantly exhausted and could barely stay awake to care for my babies, even after getting some sleep. That was until sleep disappeared entirely. My heartbeat thudded so loudly in my ears that it kept me wide awake. I could feel its deep pulsation pounding in my chest. Even then my mind still insisted, "It's all in your head."

On the day of my sons' first birthday party, I made my way up the stairs but stopped halfway to sit and rest, a routine that had become all too familiar for me. After a long and tiring day, I attempted to sleep. Lying in bed, I felt my heart racing. The pulsing and pounding in my chest drowned out everything else, as if my heart was echoing in my ears—*thump, thump*—making it feel like it was outside my body rather than deep within my chest. The sound agitated me, and I felt like I was about to jump out of my skin. I didn't know how to deal with these sensations, and once again my racing thoughts interrupted my body's signals.

This time, however, I chose to respond differently. Instead of ignoring my body, I decided to listen to it. Rather than turning away, I moved toward it. Something deep inside me urged me to listen. I placed my hands on my racing, heavy heart, resting them on my chest and focusing on the gentle pressure and warmth they provided to the thumping beneath. I noticed that the longer I kept my hands there, the slower the racing became. I embraced my body in that moment, just as I would comfort my babies when they were in distress. My touch gave me a sense of being cared for and seen in a way I hadn't experienced from anyone outside of myself. The longer I stayed with this sensation, the more information I was able to gather.

I noticed that not only was my heart pounding but I also struggled to breathe. I felt a sense of fear due to my breathlessness, but my touch provided comfort, and surprisingly the fear lessened. I remained present with my hands on my heart, and gradually my breath began to shift. Something about my touch was slowing things down and allowing me to listen in a new way, even though I didn't yet understand how. (In chapter 2 you will discover how your touch can be a powerful gift to your body's feeling of safety and security.)

After a few minutes I found that I could take deeper breaths. My breathing changed and my body felt calmer and still, even though my heart continued to race. What happened next felt natural in the moment, emerging from the immediacy of my experience. I spontaneously began a conversation with my heart, asking it what it was trying to tell me. "What do you want me to know?" It may sound odd to talk to your heart, but this is the language of embodied self-compassion that we will return to throughout this book. At that moment my words felt right; it was as if I was finally listening, and my body and I were no longer separate but together. The messages I received were clear: "Something is very wrong" and "This is not anxiety."

The next day I insisted on additional blood tests, which were initially refused. These tests revealed that I had been suffering from Graves' disease, an autoimmune condition that attacks the thyroid gland. It is often triggered by pregnancy and childbirth and is highly correlated, like many autoimmune diseases, with past trauma.[1] The overproduction of thyroid hormone in my body had become so severe that my endocrinologist informed me I was experiencing a thyroid storm, a dangerous condition. All those signals my body was sending me—symptoms that had been dismissed as stress and "new mother overload," including the nervousness and severe anxiety I felt—were manifestations of this autoimmune condition.

I felt both relieved and enraged. I recalled the many occasions when my female body was repeatedly dismissed, especially regarding my extreme weight loss. I received comments like, "Wow! You lost your baby weight so quickly; you should be happy!" and "I wish my body responded to stress that way!" These statements made me realize how women's bodies are often overlooked even as they desperately cry out for attention. I was furious with my doctors for taking so long to see and hear me, and I was equally angry with myself for not recognizing my own needs sooner.

Little did I know that I was internalizing my rage both mentally and physically. My mind was overwhelmed with thoughts about what "could've, should've, would've" happened, indicating that I was stuck in a cycle of blame, shame, and regret—which you will read about in chapter 6. This left me questioning if my condition was due to something I had done.

Then came the anger and resentment toward my body, as if it had betrayed and deceived me. A litany of thoughts paraded through my mind: "Why would you do this to me? I recovered and was treating you kindly for so many years! Why do you always turn against me? Will you ever stop burdening me? Maybe it's my fault for messing up my hormonal system in the past. You probably did this to yourself! Maybe it was all the trauma you experienced as a child!" The self-blaming thoughts went on.

Surprisingly, the rage toward myself did not last long as self-compassion rushed in to say, "But how could you have known? You were trying to listen. You did not know how!" Self-compassion, once again, produced the softening and release my body was longing for, which allowed for the vulnerable emotion of profound grief to be seen and felt. Everything felt stuck and heavy inside. I would later come to understand this internal experience as *grief stuck*, which you will learn about in chapter 6.

My endocrinologist recommended immediate radiation treatment to destroy my thyroid gland to stop my body's attack on it. I would then need to rely on synthetic hormones for the rest of my life. Self-compassion continued to provide me with the necessary softness to hold and feel the challenging emotions I was experiencing. It also helped me to grow a fierce protective instinct that kept me vigilant about my body when it needed care the most. You will learn to nurture this dual nature of self-compassion—the gentle and the fierce—in chapter 5 and understand why both are essential for building a new relationship with your body.

I made sure to nourish my body consistently and predictably, just as I did for my two babies. I remained vigilant about attending my doctor's appointments and getting blood tests, as my medications needed regular adjustments. I advocated for myself medically, persistently pursuing what I needed even when I overheard a doctor dismissively calling me "crazy" to a medical resident in training.

I wish I could say my body returned to feeling normal, but the truth is it never felt like itself again. This could be because of the missing master gland, the synthetic hormones in my system, or perhaps the trauma of being a new, young mom compounded by the strain on my marriage and my ongoing physical discomfort. I'm not sure—I just knew my body and I needed more. This realization ultimately led me to find forgiveness for my body and to deepen my understanding of myself, paving the way for embodiment.

My Return to Embodiment Through Body Forgiveness

While the experience of calming myself and my racing heart was dramatic, I first discovered the seemingly magical ability of my body to go from anxious to calm during my senior year of high school when I was required to take yoga as my gym class. I attended an all-girls Catholic high school, which seems like an unlikely place to find a yoga class, especially in the 1980s. Nevertheless, there we were. The girls in my class often complained about the teacher and the poses, and I joined them. What I didn't admit to them was how much I truly loved it. I felt incredible after each session, like something had changed within me. I could sense a different part of myself that I didn't know existed. Despite the chaos in my life and my struggles with an eating disorder, after each class I would leave feeling lighter in both mind and body. It was as if all my worries faded into the background, and I could experience a sense of connection and a feeling of being "at home." As my body calmed, I noticed that I could also slow down my mind's worries. The more my mind settled, the calmer my body became. I had no idea at the time that I was influencing and regulating the internal functioning of my nervous system—a concept that will be explored throughout this book. All I knew at seventeen was that I felt better.

After high school I stepped away from my yoga practice, but I didn't forget the internal sense of quiet, presence, and aliveness it brought me. So during my thyroid *storm*—a term that truly reflects its embodied experience—I found myself returning to yoga, seeking the safety and sense of home I'd once experienced in my body. I needed something to help me navigate the chaos.

Through the practice I began to experience what you'll discover in the somatic practices in this book: the power of pausing, slowing down, and sensing and feeling into your body. Yoga became my way to anchor myself back to my center, shifting my internal energy toward calmness and safety and awakening my body awareness. Yoga was the particular somatic method that I found, but there are many gentle movement practices that can remind you what it means to feel good.

Our bodies' internal communication takes time to develop. When I started attending class three to four days a week, the first change

I noticed was that I breathed differently. That was a cool thing to observe, as I had never paid such close attention to my breath with any consistency before. We often remain unaware of our body's automatic functions until we slowly guide our mind to pay attention to our somatic experiences. As my body awareness increased, it began to influence the way I thought.

I often showed up to class feeling awful—either overstimulated from too much thyroid hormone or sluggish from too little. This cycle continued for years as my doctors attempted to find the proper dosage. I was consumed by constant worry and frustration, wondering if I would ever feel at ease again. My preoccupation with feeling unwell filled my mind in the same way that my pounding heartbeat filled my ears. It was hard to think about anything else.

I was caught in a vicious cycle between what my body was experiencing and what my mind was telling me about what my body was experiencing—until I rolled out my mat and mindfully attended to the sensations in my body. Moving and sensing my body began to shift my mind. Neuroscience now offers a wealth of understanding about this, which you'll learn more about in chapter 3, including what a sensation is and how attending to your sensory experience helps build a lasting and forgiving relationship with your body.

In those yoga classes, the physical and emotional symptoms were still there, but for those ninety minutes my focus shifted. I was present and mindful. When we are attuned to our bodies in this way, attending to our in-the-moment experience, we are in presence with our bodies—which we'll explore further in chapter 8. Practicing presence in our bodies is a crucial step toward embodiment and learning what it means to live embodied.

On my mat I attended to every movement my body made. In yoga, especially when moving slowly and holding a pose, you have to focus. My teacher would say, "If your mind goes anywhere but this moment, you will fall." I didn't want to fall, so initially I worked hard to stay focused and present. I stopped running away from my sensations, stopped fearing, obsessing, and worrying about them. I learned to stay present to them, like when I rested my hands on my pounding heart. This presence allowed me to release the layers of tension and body armor that had built up over the years. You'll learn more about the power of staying with your body's sensory messages in chapter 9.

Through compassion and forgiveness toward my body, I came to understand that my body was doing the best it could to survive, working hard to protect me and keep me safe. As my mind released its grip, so did my body. When my body was held in safety, my emotions could flow freely. Grief turned into grieving and a new relationship between my body and me began to develop—all from learning to listen and respond to my body in a new way.

Through the practices of sensory awareness, my body received the gift of internal ease and returned to balance as best it could. Things weren't perfect. I still felt, and occasionally feel, unwell. I still struggle with body image as my body ages and changes, and I was recently diagnosed with another autoimmune disease. Despite all of that, things are quieter inside and there is less reactivity. My critical mind comes around only once in a while, and self-compassion shows up quickly to soothe it. Anger, regret, and grief toward myself and my body have been replaced by forgiveness and a deep regard, honor, and reverence for what I have learned—and continue to learn—from my body.

This is the process of body forgiveness. Through this process, I eventually came to understand, embrace, and believe that my body never meant to cause me any harm. I knew in my heart that my body didn't want any of this either. My body and mind were no longer at war, divided and disembodied; they became one. My body was no longer the enemy. For the first time, I could sense the meaning of *embodiment*, or the mind-body-spirit connection. Body forgiveness acknowledges and honors your body's innate intelligence and its longing for reconnection.

It is precisely this change that I hope you will experience in the pages of this book. Even though you may not know it yet, your body never asked for any of this pain and suffering either. It never wanted to cause you pain, betray you, or leave you feeling alone. It never meant to change, get sick, age, or stand out when all you wanted was to fit in. It never meant to scare you or make you feel unsafe. It never wanted to feel hated or unsafe.

Your body longs for the same things your mind longs for: ease, steadiness, peace, stability, homeostasis, safety, security, connection, and most of all, belonging. Your body has always been here to teach you the opposite of what you may feel toward it. It is here to teach you about forgiveness, compassion, and connection. Women, by nature, are connectors. We thrive on community and connection—with ourselves, our bodies, and one another. You are not meant to embark on this journey alone. This book is designed to be your companion along the way, a compassionate guide to lean on, especially during challenging times.

A Few Words About Words

Just as the title of this book, *Your Body Never Meant You Any Harm*, may have caused a shift within you, the words used throughout this book are intentionally chosen to do the same by centering your body as an alive, feeling, and sensing being. This is the language of embodied self-compassion. At first it may feel unfamiliar—especially if, like many of us, you have viewed your body as a separate entity, something observed rather than experienced. Yet as the title of this book suggests, words profoundly shape our bodily experience. We embody the words we use. You'll discover how the language you use each day—when talking to or about your body—can either nurture a closer relationship or create distance. Embodied self-compassion combines self-kindness with somatic awareness, guiding you to reframe challenging moments with greater compassion and mindfulness. As one of my participants shared, "You can just feel the difference in your body!"

Embodied self-compassion includes learning how to recognize and accurately assess your body's internal messages and meet them in a new, gentle way. A term you will encounter early on and throughout this book is *interoceptive awareness* (IA). *Interoception* refers to the communication we receive from within our bodies, specifically through our sensations. From the start, you will learn what a sensation is as well as how to begin to identify your own unique sensory body. Sensations reflect our body's innate intelligence and serve as its internal language, providing ongoing, moment-to-moment communication. Learning to notice, identify, listen to, and respond to this internal language is essential for establishing a new, healthy relationship with your body.

Returning to Your Body Through Practice and Reflection

This book is not just about conveying information; it is meant to offer a somatic experience. You will find practices and reflections accompanying each section that help you pause, slow down, and take your time to reconnect with your body. This approach emphasizes the importance of centering your body and its internal experiences, demonstrating that these experiences can be just as significant, if not more so, than your thoughts. The practices and reflections support you in retraining your focus on your body, guiding you back to embodied living and nurturing a new relationship with yourself. I strongly suggest doing the practices in order, as they build upon one another. I also encourage you to take as much time as you need with each practice. Healing takes time, so give yourself that gift.

Before you begin I suggest you gather the following items:

- a journal

- a pen or pencil
- a voice recorder, such as a voice memo app on your smartphone
- a pillow or cushion
- a self-massage device, such as a massage roller or trigger-point massage tool

Each chapter contains multiple practices for experiential growth. The practices are based on two different categories:

Embodied Reflections: These reflective questions are designed to enhance your self-awareness and body awareness. Take your time when writing or recording your answers and plan to revisit them. It's normal not to have immediate answers. When you return to them frequently, you may find the answers you seek or discover new insights.

Embodied Practices: These somatic practices aim to help you reconnect with your sensory experience, heightening your body awareness, interoceptive knowledge, and personal growth. Some practices invite you to reflect on words, like a mantra or a meditation. These can be helpful to voice record so that you can listen to them whenever you wish. Some of the longer practices are available as recordings on the publisher's website at www.shambhala.com /body-forgiveness-practices. I will indicate if that is the case in the introduction to each of them. I encourage revisiting the practices often, as you will come to recognize how much your body learns through repetition. Some practices ask you to make small movements. You are encouraged to modify and adapt all the practices to what feels comfortable and good for your body. Some of the practices invite you to use self-touch to enhance sensory awareness. You can use your hands or a self-massager for this purpose.

This book guides you, step by step, through the stages of body forgiveness, paving the way for true embodiment. By compassionately working with the practices, you will learn to cultivate a new and unique relationship with your body—one that is shaped by your inner wisdom and the harmony of your mind and body in the present moment. In doing so, you will return to a more embodied life and come to understand that your body truly never meant you any harm.

Reading with Compassionate Embodied Presence

Body forgiveness begins with unlearning and learning something new, which is never easy. To support this process, it will help you to read this book with attention, intention, and care. This embodied approach to reading allows you to slow down and absorb information in a present and grounded way. It is different from much of the reading we do today where we scroll and skim and rarely let things sink in.

The following tips will help you bring embodied self-compassion to your experience of reading this book, giving you the best chance for allowing the information to transform you.

1. Read each chapter slowly. Pause after each paragraph and notice how what you just read is landing inside your body. If you become tired or feel overwhelmed, this is your body's way of saying you're at capacity. Set the book aside and come back to it when you're ready.

2. Engage in the embodied reflections and practices. Take note of which ones resonate with you the most. Come back to practice those as often as you like.

3. Consider reading (or listening) during a specific time of the day that naturally feels like a more easeful time free of distractions.

4. Find a comfortable position for your body as you read (or listen), one that brings some ease to your body and supports your attention and focus.

5. Congratulate yourself for reading this way: It is your first step toward compassionately attending to and listening to your body.

Let's begin!

Understanding

i'm thinking how cruel i've been
and wondering when did i learn
to treat myself this way
who told me my body was my enemy
when did the war start
—ZOË LAWRIE

THANK YOU FOR BEING HERE. I know starting this journey is not easy, and you may wonder where to begin. We begin with a new kind of understanding. You already possess a lot of knowledge about your body and your life. This book aims to offer you a whole new perspective. Part one and its chapters explore what makes it so challenging to even imagine getting closer to your body, much less developing a deeper relationship with it. You will quickly realize that larger forces have disrupted this connection and that these influences did not originate with you. They stem from our disembodied world, making the journey back to embodiment challenging, though not impossible.

Beneath the judgments and shame you may be experiencing lies a wealth of internal sensory knowledge and protection your body has been eager to share. Although it may not feel this way right now, your body's nature is compassionate, forgiving, and designed to protect you. By the end of part one, I hope you will find renewed hope and curiosity, knowing your body has been waiting a long time for you.

1

UNDERSTANDING DISEMBODIMENT AND BODIES IN THE WORLD

Your body needs you, your feelings need you, your perceptions need you. The wounded child in you needs you. Your suffering needs you to listen and acknowledge it. Go home and be there for all these things.[1]

—THICH NHAT HANH

THE FIRST STAGE of body forgiveness begins with understanding. Have you ever wondered why so many women feel divided, conflicted, vulnerable, disconnected, or even filled with shame and blame toward their bodies? You may be one of them. You may also feel guilty and blame yourself for the disconnection with your body. Like countless other women, you may be wondering how this happened. When did this all begin and how does it continue?

This book will help you understand why disconnection from your body happens, why it persists, and what is needed to heal. This chapter introduces how and where it all began. Learning about disembodiment will clarify why so many women, like yourself, struggle to find peace, connection, and stability in and with their bodies. You are not to blame for this separation; it is not your fault. It is the result of a global problem that began long before you were born.

Each of us is on a journey to create a new relationship with our body. While our experiences of disconnection are unique, the origins are not personal. They stem from larger societal forces that have shaped how we relate to our bodies. This sense of separation stems from a collective, global experience that you deserve to understand. Acknowledging that this disconnection did not originate with you is the first step toward reconnecting with your body.

It Hasn't Been Easy to Be a Body in This World

I wish we lived in a world where we regarded bodies, especially the female body, with respect and dignity and agreed that bodies are worthy beyond their size, appearance, capability, or age. A world that honored both body and mind and believed that bodies could offer just as much (if not more) understanding as our minds. Our bodies play a vital role in informing us about our physical and mental health, yet our healthcare and mental-health systems often fail to listen to and respect this knowledge. Instead, our systems of care divide the mind and the body. At the same time, a persistent emphasis on body image—the outward appearance of our bodies—remains a primary means of validating our worth.

As the mind-body division collides with the image-obsessed world, we get pulled further away from our body's truth, its nature. The more we stray from our internal, sensory-based, intuitive understanding, the more disconnected we become from our body. As a result, our body ends up feeling like a stranger or, worse yet, our enemy. If this has happened to you, please know you are not alone.

Even though our lived experiences are different and unique, we share a universal suffering that is often referred to in self-compassion work as our common humanity. Body forgiveness honors this common humanity, acknowledging that we have all experienced some form of mind-body disconnection and that we live in a world that is often unkind and unsafe for many bodies. I wish this were not the case, but the harsh truth is that the world is often less kind and less safe for those whose bodies do not conform to culturally defined norms or standards that are deemed most valuable within the dominant cultural belief system, leading to further disconnection and division for many women.

Body disconnection is a global tragedy perceived as an individual one. When it persists throughout our lifespan, it can infiltrate our entire life and become so mentally and physically ingrained that we start to believe the thoughts we have, the feelings we experience, and the sense of disconnection and unsafety we feel in our bodies are our fault. Without comprehending the reasons behind this widespread issue, you may continue to blame yourself for the ongoing disappointment and distress you feel with your body, leading to an endless cycle of searching for what's wrong and trying to fix it. Many women find themselves trapped in an endless loop, seeking everything from the right foods and body size to optimal health, strength, energy, and the latest strategies for anti-aging or illness prevention. Even if we aren't actively seeking solutions, we are constantly bombarded with messages urging us to make our bodies desirable to others instead of focusing on what feels good for ourselves. Pause here to notice what all of this feels like inside. If you feel a sense of exhaustion, depletion, and exasperation, you are not alone.

There is nothing inherently wrong with desiring or wishing for your body to be different. However, wishing and longing for a different body is not an innate behavior—it developed over time and can be unlearned. By the end of this book, you will discover what you and your body truly desire and learn to stop searching outside yourself for answers. Instead, you will find those answers within, as you did in the beginning.

EMBODIED REFLECTION

What Do You Long For?

This meditative practice is an open inquiry for you and your body. I encourage you to reflect on the questions silently at first and then use them as a journal prompt, recording your responses in your journal or as an audio message. Ask each question three times before moving on to the next. Continue to ask the last question as many times as you'd like to allow for deeper inquiry and truth to unfold.

- Right now, what do I long for in my body?

- Right now, what do I most long for in my body?

- Right now, what do I really, most long for in my body?

- Right now, what do I really, really, most long for in my body?

Asking these questions daily can help you stay connected to the essence of what you long for. Discovering through embodiment feels different—you are no longer searching for answers elsewhere but rather returning home to your body and its truth. There is no more questioning. Instead, there is a mindful, awake, and aware listening that arises from your internal body's truth. The unfortunate reality is that, despite being born connected to your body's truth, you lost this connection along the way. What we truly desire is reconnection.

When Mind and Body Became Strangers

To understand how we lost touch with the nature of our bodies, we need to look back in time to a cultural paradigm, established long before we were born, that dramatically altered our perception of all bodies and affected our inherent natural connection with them. This paradigm, known as the mind-body divide, or dualism, spread across the Western world in the seventeenth century and has since permeated the globe, evolving into a worldview that keeps us separated from our most natural relationship with our bodies.

Dualism, also known as the Cartesian split, is attributed to the French philosopher René Descartes, widely known for his declaration "I think, therefore I am" (*Cogito, ergo sum*). Descartes' theory proposed that the mind (or soul) and the body are fundamentally different substances: The mind is immaterial and responsible for thought, while the body is material and operates according to physical laws. This dualistic perspective influenced philosophers and scientists who were debating whether human identity is rooted in the mind, the body, or both.

Prior to the seventeenth century, bodies were viewed as spiritual entities. Bodies were believed to be a connected informative source of sensation, reason, and wisdom, with the soul or spirit within the body seen as the motivating force behind physiological functions, cognition, and reasoning. This perspective aligned with ancient spiritual traditions and Indigenous cultures worldwide. Because of this interconnected view, it was considered essential to keep the human body intact so the soul could ascend to heaven. This belief posed a significant conflict for the advancement of modern science: How could one cut open, dissect, explore, and investigate a body without disturbing the soul if they were viewed as one?

Mind-body dualism was seen as a solution, allowing the study of the body to move beyond the ethical constraints imposed by the Catholic Church. With this new belief, scientists could examine and observe the body without fearing disruptions to the soul, as the mind and body were declared fundamentally different and unable to exist in unity. The mind was considered an immaterial thinking substance, while the body was seen as a material unthinking substance—two separate and independent realms. This belief placed greater value on the mind, and bodies were stripped of their inherent qualities, such as spirit and nature. This reductionist perspective not only shaped the thinking of Descartes' time but also marked a worldwide paradigm shift contributing to the view of bodies as objects to observe and control rather than as living, feeling, spiritual, sensory beings that embody our identity.

Your Mind Over Your Body

We have all been taught to value our thinking mind over our sensing, feeling body. This reflection invites you to consider how entrenched this belief is for you.

- Do I believe I can know myself only through my mind?

- Do I believe my body has anything to offer me in the way of self-knowledge or telling me what it needs?

- Do I believe I can resolve my problem with my body through my mind?

There are no right or wrong answers to these questions. They are meant to help you get curious about whether you value your mind over your body and to consider if there might be a different way.

Moving Beyond Body Objectification

Viewing your body as an object is a direct result of the dualistic, reductionist view that encourages us to observe and treat our bodies as objects instead of as intimate parts of ourselves. It encourages us to believe that our self-identity and knowledge are isolated in our minds and thoughts and separated from our sensing bodies. It robs us of the ability to trust our bodies to communicate with us and help us feel safe and empowered with a sense of agency, and it leaves us with a profound sense of separation.

This dualistic paradigm is inherent in much of contemporary scientific thought, influencing our medical and mental-health systems. It forms the foundation of the biomedical model in medicine and shapes our perception of disease. In this view, disease in the body is seen as a deviation from the norm, fostering the belief that we can control our health and well-being through effort and by continually seeking out new solutions. This perspective promotes the idea that health and well-being should be attainable for everyone, yet it fails to acknowledge that health unfolds differently for each individual. Moreover, it overlooks the fact that physical and mental health are privileges not everyone has access to and are impacted by factors such as gender, sexual orientation, age, disability status, socioeconomic status, and geographic location.

Neuroscience, trauma research, and consciousness studies now validate and respect what the great mystics, Indigenous cultures, yogis, and spiritual teachers of the past have long understood: Our bodies and minds are deeply interconnected. Despite this understanding, the concept of "mind over body" still prevails, and body knowledge remains undervalued in medicine and mental health. The belief of mind over body is entrenched in our medical and mental-health systems, which value cognitive and behavioral treatments as the standards of care and best practices for all mental-health concerns. In research, we continue to value numerical data over the lived experience of a human.

At the same time, somatic therapies remain on the sidelines as alternative treatments despite new scientific knowledge confirming the central role somatic processes play in self-development and internal health. The mind-body divide has become entrenched as a paradigm in contemporary culture and the medical system. The weight and healthcare blogger Ragen Chastain uses the term *paradigm entrenchment* when discussing the ingrained fat bias and weight stigma present in our medical system and healthcare practices that remain entrenched in the minds of the majority despite known evidence to the contrary. Chastain asks, "What if there might be something I could learn that is different from what I have believed until now?"[2] Unfolding the developmental stages of body forgiveness will help you shift from viewing your body as just an object to living in connection with your body, yourself, and others in a new way.

From Disembodiment to Diet Culture

Disembodiment is a phenomenon that affects everyone, regardless of gender identity. However, women have disproportionately felt its impact, largely because of the pervasive influence of diet culture. Diet culture is so ingrained in women's lives that choosing not to participate can often lead to feelings of isolation and a sense of not belonging. Pause to consider how radical it would be to be a woman who eats freely in front of other women, does not shame or blame her body, and does not buy into the next diet or weight-manipulation technique. It's not easy to stand up against the majority. The diet industry, which is estimated to be worth over sixty-six billion dollars, thrives on women's feelings of disconnection and shame about their bodies.[3]

While the origins of the mind-body division predate diet culture, this oppressive system has thrived in the environment created by that division. It encourages the belief that our minds and bodies are separate entities rather than the deeply connected partners they truly are. This misconception allows diet culture to continue to gain power, keeping women disembodied and unaware of their own bodies. This system *relies* on you remaining disembodied so that it may continue to exist.

Diet culture fosters the false belief that we can connect with our bodies and belong in the world only by changing our body size to conform to unattainable images and ideals. Women often engage in futile efforts to control the size of their bodies, which is precisely what this predatory system wants: to keep us coming back for more. Relying on an external system to tell you what you and your body need arises from the lack of trust that disembodiment creates. This disconnection is most clearly expressed through our obsession with and focus on body image. The more you disconnect from your internal body, the more you try to define and connect with yourself through image, or what I call the surface body. This leads to a constant state of comparison and judgment of yourself and other women. If you identify with this cycle, know that you are not alone. The more we focus on image, the further we drift from becoming embodied—and the more the external system thrives.

Christy Harrison, an anti-diet dietitian, defines diet culture as a system that oppresses bodies by glorifying thinness, assigning higher value and health to certain body sizes over others, and reinforcing fatphobia.[4] This system has affected us all, as well as our female ancestors before us. Think back to your mother, possibly even your grandmother and great-grandmother. How present was this system in their lives? How present is it in yours?

No body is exempt from scrutiny in this system; however, women's bodies have historically been the most influenced and manipulated, particularly large-bodied women and women of color. In her book *Fearing the Black Body: The Racial Origins of Fatphobia*, Professor Sabrina Strings explores the racial origins of fatphobia. She highlights how fatphobia has its roots in the Transatlantic slave trade, during which time colonists equated superiority, morality, and value with the white body and promoted body restraint and thinness as expressions of this superiority. As a result, fat became associated with racial inferiority and immorality.[5] Stigma based on gender and weight is not in your imagination—it is all around us.

The Dangers of Weight and Health Bias

Weight bias is a widespread form of prejudice that is harmful both mentally and physically to people whose bodies are perceived to have excess adipose tissue, also known as fat, increasing stigmatization. The damaging belief that individuals who are in a larger body lack willpower or are lazy perpetuates the misconception that body weight is entirely within an individual's control and that any excess weight or weight change that moves the number on the scale higher results from individual choices and can be reversed easily. This keeps the burden on the individual rather than on examining the political, social, and cultural systems that drive these beliefs. These antiquated views of body size perpetuate fat bias and the fear of fat, leading women to extreme behaviors to control their body weight at any cost in the name of health and wellness.

The National Eating Disorders Association (NEDA) highlights a strong connection between weight stigma and chronic dieting, which can lead to disordered eating and eating disorders.[6] Chronic dieting is an attempt to shrink one's body to fit societal standards of acceptance and belonging. It often results in a harmful disconnection from one's body. As the author and activist Sonia Renee Taylor notes in her book *The Body Is Not an Apology*, a healthcare system that stigmatizes weight perpetuates the predatory nature of diet culture by instilling and reinforcing shame and bias.[7]

We live in a world where women's bodies get attention for their external appearance while little focus is given to our internal needs. This remains apparent in healthcare and medical research. A report from the World Economic Forum and the McKinsey Health Institute states that women spend 25 percent more of their lives in poor health than men, and yet in nearly three-quarters of cases where a disease predominantly affects women, funding still favors males. Moreover, research into diseases impacting men are overfunded while those affecting women are underfunded.[8] The researcher Lisa Bowleg points out that women of color face even greater health disparities: They experience higher disease prevalence, lower survival rates, and more severe illness earlier in life compared to white women and men yet continue to encounter significant inequities in public-health resources.[9]

What Do You Notice Now?

Take a moment to notice what's happening inside you after reading the information about body stigma and diet culture. Understanding the hidden agenda of diet culture is a challenging task. As you start to look beyond the veiled manipulations of diet culture, various sensations, feelings, and thoughts may emerge. Notice them arise and gently respond, *No wonder this has been so hard.*

Claiming Your Right to Embodiment

If your body does not fit into the socially constructed norms and dominant value systems of your society, you are more likely to experience the shared suffering of disembodiment and have additional layers of suffering. If your body is light-skinned, smaller in size, heterosexual, cisgender, perceived as healthy and functional in movement and ability, stable in mental health and neurotypical, aging well, and is not yet sick or old, your path to reembodiment is likely to be easier. This may be difficult to accept, but it is a reality in our world.

If your body is deemed nonbelonging according to the cultural standard of the time and its systems, the path of body forgiveness and embodiment will be more challenging. There will be more suffering along the way. I am sorry about this. Please know that I don't pretend to know your lived experience. I only know my own and the thousands of stories I have heard and held for over thirty-five years. I have been, and still am, in a body that fits into societal standards, which allows me to belong in the world with relative ease. I am thin, able-bodied, neurotypical, cisgender, and heterosexual. As a teenager, even when I struggled with an eating disorder, I could hide my suffering. Even as my body withered away, it was celebrated, desired, and envied by my friends and other women. Despite my struggles, these privileges allowed my journey back to reembodiment to be more accessible than it may be for many of you.

Throughout more than three decades as a clinician, I have witnessed clients who live in larger bodies struggle to live embodied in a world that fights against their very existence. Please understand that the path to embodiment is still yours to have. Reconnecting with your body is your right, and it is something your body deeply longs for. It is disheartening that these prescriptive systems and messages still exist, exerting relentless pressure to manipulate, control, and shame you into submission and disembodiment. While the path to embodiment will be challenging, I can promise you that as you learn to reembody, you will experience greater internal empowerment and connection, no matter your size, shape, or abilities. The more internal power and connection you develop, the more capable you will feel about engaging with the world—standing up to, speaking out against, and challenging the systems that aim to disembody us. Through the stages of body forgiveness, we will learn together that embodiment is our superpower against these systems, allowing us to establish stronger boundaries, foster protection, and build resilience.

But there is work to do. By *work*, I don't mean the type of work you may be used to. I don't mean striving, pushing, or grasping. I mean the work it takes to develop a gentle and compassionate understanding of what led you so far away from yourself and the common humanity that reminds us we are not alone.

When You Are Body Shamed

Stigmatization induces shame both within our self-identity and in our physical bodies. I will say more about this in chapter 6, where we will examine shame in depth. For now, this reflection is meant to offer you a new perspective on what body stigmatization and shame have done and continue to do to your relationship with your body. Please note that this reflection is open to all forms of what is perceived as body stigmatization. I encourage you to journal about the following questions:

- After I experience a body-shaming moment out in the world, what happens to my relationship with my body?

- Do I feel closer to it or further away from it?

- Do I want to care for my body more or less?

- Do I comfort myself and my body, or do I further shame and punish my body? Body shame typically leads to further shame, blame, and disembodiment, so don't feel bad if that is how you answered. How could it not?

- Pause, and place a hand on your heart. Say silently or out loud, *But how could I not!*

How could you *not* get swept away by diet culture's manipulations? How could you *not* blame and shame yourself and maybe even others? How could you *not* seek out maladaptive behaviors to adapt to a disembodied world? You were never the cause of your shame. Instead, you absorbed shame from the outside, which landed inside. Once shame is internalized, it creates a perpetual cycle—a search for validation that attempts to fix, improve, or make yourself acceptable. This internalized shame continues to damage the already fragile relationship between you and your body. No one is born hating or shaming their body or anyone else's. No one. Please use these simple yet powerful words throughout the day whenever you experience a moment of shame or stigma.

Why We Learned to Fear and Control Our Bodies

Can you remember back to a time in childhood when you moved through the world without feeling anxious about your body? For some of you, this may be a distant memory, but many of you won't be able to recall a time when you didn't experience body anxiety. I define *body anxiety* as the ruminating thoughts and overall feeling of unease around our culture's obsession with beauty standards and thinness. If body anxiety goes unnoticed and unaddressed, it can become pervasive, leaving your mind and body in a state of distress and dysregulation, which we will discuss in chapter 4. It's important to remember that you were not born with body anxiety. Sandra Lee Bartky, an influential feminist philosopher in the 1990s, purported that the compulsion of equating thinness to beauty has never been an individual pathology but is a result of an "entrenched cultural anxiety," an anxiety that has spread across the globe.[10]

Our connection to our bodies is eroding across cultures as dominant practices and beliefs continue to dictate how bodies should look and behave. In my training and teaching experience in embodiment, I have witnessed this entrenched anxiety impact many women, even those from cultures where such anxieties were once absent, leading to a disconnection from their heritage and cultural practices, as well as the sense of community and wholeness that these once provided. Many share how they have distanced themselves from childhood foods that once felt connecting and supportive but now induce shame and embarrassment. This shift results from dominant cultural ideals that lead them to believe their traditional practices are wrong, unhealthy, or excessive for their bodies. Pulling away from what once felt nurturing and safe can leave you increasingly insecure and fearful of your body, vulnerable to the external influences of diet culture.

Many years ago, while working on my doctoral dissertation on the role that self-compassion played in eating-disorder recovery, I came across a fascinating yet disturbing book called *Holy Anorexia* by Rudolf Bell that offered a critical perspective missing from our understanding of women's bodies and the search for meaning. As early Eastern religions adopted the belief in the duality of body and mind, the practice of restraining bodily desires to achieve purity and closeness to the divine became common. Christian saints, like many early ascetics in Eastern religions, endured fasting and suppressed physical urges and feelings as a way to seek enlightenment. Many starved themselves to death in an attempt to move closer to the spirit and free the body to allow the soul to commune with God. Their motivation was spiritual practice. However, Bell hypothesizes that these saints may have also been conforming to the patriarchal social structure of medieval Catholicism that defined suppressive behaviors as saintly rather than unwell.[11] In our time, diet-culture messages have become the new demigods, inviting women to suppress, deny, and withhold bodily needs and desires as a sign of superiority, willpower, and strength—when all along we have been searching for safety, agency, and power within our bodies. Whenever we deny and deprive ourselves of what we need on any level, we leave our bodies confused and powerless, and we reinforce the belief that body-based needs and desires are somehow wrong, shameful, unnatural, and need to be dampened and controlled.

As a small child, I loved to eat, and I indulged in food freely. However, in high school, friends and classmates teased me about my size and my appetite, especially those who were withholding food from themselves. I became confused about the impulses of my body and came to believe that I was supposed to suppress my appetite despite my body's natural longing to eat.

When I was sixteen and my father passed away suddenly and traumatically, confusion about my body combined with the grief of early parental loss and the raging diet-culture messages of the 1980s led me down the same path as many of you. I came to believe the solution was to deprive my body of nourishment and desire by focusing outward on body image rather than inward on what I needed most—feeling my grief and receiving nurturing, connected, compassionate care.

How Long Has It Been?

Respecting your body's needs and desires is central to the sense of belonging and embodiment we all long for. Consider the following questions to explore how long you have felt confusion about your body's needs.

- How long have you and your body been confused? How long have you denied your body's needs: food, hunger and fullness cues, rest and activity, connection and care, pleasure?

- How many of the women in your life who came before you— mother, grandmother, aunts, sisters—did you observe in this same state of confusion and denial of their bodies' needs and desires?

Denying Your Needs Leads to Body Confusion

If you have found yourself confused about your body's needs— denying them, not knowing how to be with them, and placing others' needs above yours—you are not alone. Generation after generation of women have learned to deny their bodies' needs. For centuries, female bodies have carried the wounds of disembodiment, resulting in confusion, shame, blame, and self-criticism. Joan, one of the study participants, said, "I needed to know what imprinted inside me, because that impacted me and left me feeling like I never had a day of love for my body."

The psychologist Marcia Germaine Hutchinson, who wrote about our culture's influence on body-image disturbance in the 1980s, argued that the true nature of a woman's body—intuitively connected to nature, emotions, cooperation, affiliation, and community—finds little room in a patriarchal and capitalistic system. Throughout history, women and women's bodies have been seen as the "mistress of the dark," the dark being a mysterious and powerful realm of the flesh associated with instinct, irrationality, unpredictability, sensuality, uncleanliness, and evil.[12]

Although some things have improved for some women, feelings of body confusion have remained consistent. If you are one of the women still caught in this cycle, I understand. I was once in your shoes. Please remember that feelings of shame, self-blame, and self-criticism stem from wounds that were embedded in womankind long before you came into existence. If left unchecked, they can cause deeper wounds that get unknowingly passed down through generations. The cycle of shame and self-blame can lead you to believe that you are responsible for these issues, but it is important to recognize that denying your body's nature is not an individual problem—it never belonged to you or your body to begin with.

Rebuilding Your Relationship with Food

In writing a book about embodiment and the journey toward reembodiment, I cannot overlook one of the most crucial relationships that supports each stage of body forgiveness: your relationship with food. In our diet-obsessed culture, food is often the first basic need that women choose to withhold from themselves. This withholding may occur consciously or, more commonly, unconsciously. Restriction has become such a widely accepted and even celebrated practice for women that we often fail to recognize when we are denying ourselves food or not adequately meeting our body's nutritional needs.

The unfortunate reality is that many women feel excluded from the tribe if they are not engaging in some form of food restriction, dieting, shaming, or apologizing to themselves or others about their body image or food choices. Many female clients express that in a group of women, if they are not criticizing or complaining about their body size or the foods they eat, they do not feel a sense of belonging.

Your Body and Food

Reflect on the following questions in your journal or by making an audio recording of your thoughts.

- In just a few words, describe your body's current relationship with food—not a past or future relationship, but the one your body has with food right now.

- Look at the words you wrote in response to the previous question. Do they sound familiar? Is this a longstanding way you describe your relationship with food?

- Consider the first time you learned that you should eat less as a woman. When was it? What was the external message, obvious or subtle, influencing you to believe this?

- Have you ever wondered if the way you have been feeding your body is natural to your body?

- Have you ever wondered if your body knows a different way to be with food?

These critical questions invite you to be curious about your body's relationship with food and, more important, invite you to consider whether there might be a different approach. In chapter 2 you will explore the origins of your relationship with food and discover how your body longs for an opportunity to start anew, to build a new relationship with food.

Grounding into Your Needs

This practice is available as an audio recording at www.shambhala .com/body-forgiveness-practices. I invite you to explore where need originates in your body. The felt sense of a need begins at the "root" of your body. In yoga therapy this is known as your root chakra, which is located at the base of your tailbone, at your perineum and the bottom of your pelvic floor. This practice will help you connect with the origins of your body's needs and how they continue today.

1. Sit in a chair in an upright position with your feet touching the ground.

2. Press your feet into the ground and breathe in through your nose and out through your mouth. Take several breaths this way.

3. With your next breath, gently rock your pelvis forward and backward a few times. As you rock forward, your lower back will shift away from the back of the chair. As you rock backward, your lower back will shift toward the chair.

4. Now find a position that's in the middle—not too far forward and not too far backward. Stay here for a couple of breaths.

5. Imagine that the base of your tailbone grows roots every time you respond to a need that your body has. Even if you have met only a few of your body's needs today, you are rooting down to grow.

6. Envision what supports the roots as they grow. Do you see a certain color? Is there supportive ground beneath you, such as dirt, moss, or sand? If a supportive image comes to you, let it emerge. Otherwise, stay with the felt sense of roots extending down from your root chakra.

7. Say to yourself, *Sensing and attending to my body's needs roots me.*

Use this practice throughout the day to envision what your body may need. Relearning how to feel and sense these needs helps you to reconnect to your body.

Releasing Old Stories, Welcoming New Possibilities

As you reach the end of this chapter, remember that the struggles you feel in your relationship with your body are not yours alone. They are the result of powerful cultural myths and intergenerational patterns—stories about bodies, worth, and belonging that have been passed down and reinforced over centuries. These beliefs are woven into families, communities, and entire societies, shaping how we see ourselves and one another. Recognizing that your disconnection from your body is rooted in these larger forces—not personal failure— is the first step toward compassion and change.

To help clear some of the energy these old stories may have stirred, I invite you to try the "ha" breath. Inhale deeply through your nose, then exhale through your mouth with a forceful "ha" sound, releasing tension and letting go of what no longer serves you. You can return to this breath whenever you need to reset and reconnect. As you move forward, know that you are not alone on this path. Each breath, each act of curiosity or kindness toward your body, helps break the cycle and opens the possibility for healing—both for yourself and for those who come after you.

I'm just a person understanding.
—LISA, STUDY PARTICIPANT

2

UNDERSTANDING EMBODIMENT

Meeting Your Body for the First Time

Let's connect with the sense of aliveness in this body.
Breathing, pulsating, this amazing piece of nature.[1]
—**NIKKI MIRGHAFORI**

THE SECOND STAGE of body forgiveness is understanding embodiment. Now that you have explored disembodiment, it's time to shift to the purpose of this book—embodiment. This chapter invites you to revisit your origins, going back to your birth and even before. You will discover what felt most natural to your body long before separation and disembodiment occurred. You can view this chapter as a meeting with your body for the first time, an opportunity to relearn and regain what has been lost.

Your Body's First Language Is Compassion

It may be hard to believe that there was a time long ago—perhaps even before you can remember—when you were fully embodied. You were completely present and connected to each sensory experience. You felt every movement your body made, sensed your external surroundings, and noticed how they felt inside. This occurred long before you or anyone around you had any thoughts about your body.

Your body is inherently compassionate. It aims to heal and strives for homeostasis and balance. One organ supports another. By nature, your body is intimately connected within itself, and you were once compassionately connected to it even without realizing it. Thich Nhat Hanh beautifully expressed how compassion is inherent to our bodies if we pay attention. He noted that if we step on a nail, our hand instinctively reaches down to comfort our foot. Without thought, your body's natural reaction is to care for and alleviate suffering from one part to another.[2] We are born with the instinct to relieve our body's distress. This phenomenon is evident in a baby who instinctively cries in response to its own discomfort. It is the essence of self-compassion, which begins and resides within your body.

Your Body's Original Way of Knowing

At one time, you were deeply attuned to what your body was communicating—its unique signals. Before thoughts and words took over, you instinctively responded to your body's needs. Within you lies an intricate and distinct language that tells you exactly what you need for your well-being. There was a period when you understood those messages, instinctively knowing how to nurture yourself and what made you feel safe and connected. You recognized the sensations of nourishment in your body, knowing when you had enough to eat or when you needed more. You were aware of when you felt unwell and when you felt good. You also knew what brought you ease, comfort, and contentment.

Even at the molecular level, the female body demonstrates remarkable communication in choosing what it wants and needs, beginning with conception. Research shows conception is not passive; rather, it occurs through a dialogue between the mother's egg and the father's sperm as the egg releases chemical signals called chemoattractants to attract specific sperm. The Swedish researcher John Fitzpatrick, who studies reproductive behavior and evolution, has revealed that the female body can discern and select which sperm will fertilize the egg.[3] In this way, your body possesses an innate power to communicate and choose what it wants and needs—even before birth.

At first, as you were developing, you didn't have a fully formed awareness of a distinct self. Instead, all communication originated from your body. This deep-rooted communication, originating only through your somatosensory system, functioned even before birth and evolved as you grew. Your somatosensory system is a complex network of nerves that senses and gathers information about both your surroundings and your internal state. This remarkable system has been with you since the womb, serving as the first language and form of communication between you and your body.

Before I Was Born: A Journey Within

Keep your journal close and allow your imagination to come alive for this reflection that aims to help you explore your earliest body movements and sensitivity, spark your curiosity, and provide you with new insights about your body's history.

Read through the following instructions. Close your eyes or look away from the book to reflect on each question. At the end of the practice, open your eyes and quickly write about your experience to capture your immediate responses.

- Find a comfortable position either sitting or lying down. Your eyes can be closed or softly opened as you reflect.

- Gently count down, with each breath, from twenty to one.

- Imagine you are looking into the past and can see your developing self before you were born.

- Was your body moving? Was it resting? Was it stretched out long? Was it curled up?

- Were there sounds or noises you imagine you heard? Some that you liked? Some that you did not like?

- Was there a motion you imagined you liked? Motion that you did not like?

- Do you imagine your body was sensitive and perceptive? If so, what do you imagine it was noticing, sensing, and feeling?

- As this first language and communication developed, what do you imagine your body sensed then? If it could speak, what do you imagine your developing, sensing, feeling body would have said then?

This may initially seem like an unusual reflection, but engaging in this reflective practice is the essential first step toward recognizing your body for what it truly is: a sensing, feeling, living, and communicative system. Taking this perspective will shift your focus away from external judgments about body image and foster a deeper sensory understanding of your body.

I encourage you to be curious about what you imagined. Some of what you envisioned may relate to your own knowledge about your body, some might come from information others have shared with you, and some could be what you hoped your experience would be like. All these aspects are valuable and important to acknowledge.

When I was about five years old, I was told that I moved around a lot in my mother's womb. As a child, I loved moving my body, especially in any swaying, rocking, or swinging motion. I'm unsure if this is how I moved in the womb, but I like to imagine this was so. One of my earliest memories of movement was rocking on a metal rocking horse that bounced up and down and rocked back and forth. If I consider now what kind of movement I enjoy most in my body this many decades later, it is still this free-flowing, swaying and rocking motion. This is, in part, why yoga appeals to me: It feels fluid and gentle and speaks to the part within me that was in touch with this kind of movement from the start. This was the kind of movement I liked best long before I could even put words to it.

My three children were uniquely different in their body movements. My twin sons each had their own embodied expression in the womb. One stretched out long. The other curled up in a ball. Throughout their childhoods, I observed them sleeping this way. One didn't mind loud noises. The other did. My daughter was very still in the womb, so still that the doctors were concerned about her well-being. (She was fine.) Even now, at twenty-four, she does not like a lot of movement in her body and never has. She also feels her emotions intensely and expressively. I have a mother's intuition that she felt a great deal before she was born as well.

I also remember being a sensitive child. I was keenly aware of what was happening around me and could feel events viscerally within my body very quickly, although I did not know what they meant. I only knew that my body shifted inside each time something shifted on the outside. When I do this practice, I imagine I was the same in the womb. I imagine my growing body could sense and feel what was happening around me. I imagine my developing body would probably have said, "I sense tension, sadness, and lots of worry out there; rocking and swaying and moving calms that down."

You can revisit these reflection questions multiple times to observe what stays the same and what begins to change.

Your Body Is Always with You

My favorite definition of *embodiment* comes from the twentieth-century French philosopher Maurice Merleau-Ponty, who introduced a different perspective on the relationship between body and mind, one that countered the dualistic approach of Descartes. He describes the body as a living, attentive "body subject" rather than simply an object. According to Merleau-Ponty, our body is a constant presence—an ever-with-us perception. This essential understanding does not suggest that the body leads us or that we lead our body; rather, it emphasizes that our body is always a "presence" alongside us.[4]

Many of my study participants and clients, when they discuss what embodiment means to them, also refer to the idea of being present with themselves (we'll explore this topic more in part three). Unbeknownst to them, Merleau-Ponty had used the term *presence* to describe embodiment many years prior. *Presence* signifies an act of "being beside." It implies being with or next to and having an internal, felt sense of connection. This understanding of presence means that even if you forget about your body, your body never forgets you. It is always there, alongside you, connected to you, and waiting for you to recognize it with the compassion it deserves.

The Thinking Mind Over the Sensing Body

Merleau-Ponty's definition of *embodiment* challenges the dualistic, detached, and objectified perspective that views the body as separate from the self. This perspective inaccurately separates our concept of self and life from our bodily experiences and implies that the body cannot perceive experiences or events. Classical psychology and talk therapy tend to support this dualistic view, encouraging us to disregard bodily experiences or, when they are acknowledged, to convert them into objective knowledge (coming from outside of your body) through rational thought and behavior rather than through sensing what's happening inside your body. In this framework, the mind is seen as ruling over the body, despite the understanding that our body, not our mind, is the primary recipient of experiences both before and after our birth.

Our lived experiences are not merely perceived and stored in our minds, they are received and remembered by our bodies first.

Our bodies play a crucial role in helping our minds process these experiences through an intricate internal sensory communication system that functions in a continuous feedback loop between the body and the brain and nervous system. This means that at any given moment, our bodies are constantly attempting to communicate with us through sensory cues. Our challenge is that we were never taught how to listen to these signals.

Instead we were conditioned, or trained, to think more rather than experience more. Merleau-Ponty viewed the body as a source of sensory wonder and a field of awareness. He believed that our perceptions and thoughts are formed through the interplay between our sensing bodies and the entities around us—our environment and others. He suggested we are in an ongoing exchange, a constant dialogue and awareness between our body, self, environment, and others.

Merleau-Ponty also considered our bodily experiences as integral to our consciousness. We cannot separate our physical experiences from the beliefs and ideas we hold in our minds. When we learn to listen to our bodily experiences and develop an awareness and understanding of our sensing, feeling bodies, we begin to feel more connected within ourselves and with others, and the separation of mind and body dissolves. As Merleau-Ponty suggests, our bodies become the means through which we relate to all things, leading us to a fuller, richer, and more vibrant life—one that actively engages with our surroundings. It also encourages us to view our bodies not as separate entities but as an essential part of who we are, bringing us back to our true nature and the embodied experience we had before we were born.[5]

Sensory Wonderment

Embodiment starts with the possibility of experiencing something new and different. You are and have always been what Merleau-Ponty called a "sensory wonderment."[6] This practice will help you access a sense of wonder, surprise, fascination, amazement, and awe. This practice is available as an audio recording at www.shambhala.com/body-forgiveness-practices.

1. Close your eyes or keep them open and maintain a soft, resting gaze.

2. Picture yourself as a newborn baby. If you can recall a photograph of your young self, you can use that image.

3. In your mind's eye, admire that small body. Marvel at how your organs, soft skin, bones, muscles, and joints were carefully developed and how these systems learned to work together and grow. Reflect with wonder on how your body, as tiny as it is, knows how to keep all its complex systems in balance without a thought.

4. Open your eyes and look at your present-day self from your feet up. Although you may get caught up in evaluating your clothes, your body, or your self-image, recognize that underneath this distraction your natural body is still working hard every day to regain and rebalance all of your systems into a state of equilibrium called homeostasis.

5. Close your eyes again or resume your soft, resting gaze. Consider how babies investigate their bodies. They wiggle and move their hands and feet, fingers and toes. They stare in amazement and wonder, subconsciously attempting to figure out how these body parts move and how they work together. They are feeling their way into themselves.

6. Open your eyes again and look at your hands and feet. Although you may not see this right now, you once stared at them with a baby's innocent amazement and wonder.

7. Close your eyes again or resume your soft, resting gaze. Imagine a baby as she learns to roll over, scoot, crawl, and stand. Consider the amazement babies often express when they do one of these acts, perhaps finding themselves in a new spot without any idea of how their body got them there.

8. Open your eyes and gently move your body in whatever way feels enjoyable to you.

Although you may not feel it right now, you once moved with a sense of great fascination and surprised satisfaction, embodying awe with every movement you made. I encourage you to revisit this practice as often as you wish. It will help you learn to connect with the sense of wonder as our natural birthright. Each day offers an opportunity to improve how you see, look, and feel about your body.

What Your Body Knew First

You developed and entered the world deeply connected to your body, in intimate communication with it. From the moment you were born, you engaged with the world around you with sensory wonder. As your somatosensory system continued to develop, your senses of smell, taste, hearing, sight, and touch awakened in unique ways and to varying degrees. Your sense of touch developed first, around week eight of gestation, and it is the most developed sense at birth. Working with your sense of touch now is your first step toward getting to know your sensory body.

Discovering Your Relationship to Your Sense of Touch

This reflection will take you on an imaginative journey to explore the first and most prominent sense organ you were born with: your sense of touch. As you consider the following questions, you may recall memories of yourself as an infant or child. If you don't, that isn't a problem—use your imagination to deduce what the answer might be based on your current preferences. There is no right or wrong answer to these questions. Just respond to them quickly without too much thought. Taken as a whole, they will help you start to explore your relationship to the sense of touch.

- Were you the kind of infant or baby who liked to be wrapped and swaddled?

- Do you like being wrapped up or swaddled now? For example, do you enjoy weighted blankets? Or does tightly wrapping a towel or blanket around you help you relax? Do you like cuddling?

- Were you the kind of infant or baby who enjoyed being held close, heart to heart, or did you prefer to be held not so tightly so you could look out into the world?

- Do you like deep, heart-to-heart hugs now? Cuddling? Spooning? Or do you prefer something different, like just holding hands or sitting beside someone?

- Were you the kind of infant or baby who liked to be rocked or bounced up and down?

- Do you like soft, rhythmic movements now, like in yoga, dance, tai chi, or qigong? Or do you prefer high-impact movements like weightlifting, running, Pilates, stretching, or sports?

- Were you the kind of infant or baby who liked water? Did you enjoy baths, pools, lakes, or other bodies of water? Did you enjoy being under the water or only above it? Did you like the water hot, cold, warm, or cool?

- Do you like water now? Do you take baths, like to swim, or surf in the ocean? Do you enjoy being under the water or only above it? How about the temperature of the water?

These questions may seem unusual but they will help you develop an understanding of the tactile preferences of your body. The more you explore what appeals to you and your body, the deeper your relationship with it will become, allowing you to reconnect with its inherent communication signals. Considering these questions will also help you learn to recognize sensations around another key area—hunger, food, and nourishing yourself.

Food Isn't Just Nourishing, It's Nurturing

Like your sense of touch, your initial experience of nourishment also began in the womb, where your body received essential nutrients through the placenta. Your birth mother didn't have to know or think about how this happened; it simply did. Your body's initial experience with food was one of ease, contentment, and freedom. Just as you were born with an innate awareness of your somatic experience, there was a time—long before conscious thought—when you instinctively knew when you needed nourishment and how many nutrients were necessary to feel satisfied and cared for.

Yes, cared for, because food is not just about sustenance, it is also about feeling nurtured.

I understand that the words *nurture* and *food* may evoke strong reactions for some of you. If this is the case, it's important to recognize that these feelings stem from the distorted beliefs about food and bodies that have led you far away from what is most natural for your body. If you felt a reaction to these words, take a deep breath. I invite you to engage with the following reflection, which will help you rediscover your body's natural relationship with food.

Imagining Food in a New Way

This reflection allows the opportunity to imagine your relationship with food in a new way. Please reflect upon each step and journal or record your responses.

- Close your eyes or keep them slightly open with a soft, resting gaze.

- Imagine traveling back to when you were in the womb. Imagine sensing your body floating, rocking, swaying. Muted sounds around you. You didn't feel hungry because there was food ever present, coming to you through your birth mother's body. There was no thought about it, no planning, no worries, no fear. It was easy and free, leaving you in a state of contentment, rest, and nourishment that allowed your body to grow and thrive.

- Imagine how being fed this way felt nurturing to your body.

- Imagine if food could be that way for you now.

In our diet-obsessed culture, it can be hard to imagine this or to stop the reflection there. You may have the impulse to create a plan or figure out how to achieve this state. But you don't have to know anything special or do anything about this right now. All you have to do is imagine the way it once was and be curious about how your daily interactions with food would change if it were this way now.

From Innocence to Othering: When the Body Becomes a Stranger

Things have not been easy between you and your body, possibly for a long time—perhaps for as long as you can remember. Many of you likely feel that you have never been embodied or in touch with the true nature of your body, and some of you may be thinking, "I don't even know what that means." Some of you could tell me the moment when you felt this disconnection occur, while many others tell me, "This is just how it has always been between me and my body. I know nothing else." Regardless of your experience, as you learned in chapter 1, we were all born into a world that disconnected us from our body. Whether the disruption happened long ago or more recently, what matters now for healing to take place is understanding how things have been since then.

Disruption in embodiment occurs when we shift our attention from our internal sensations to the external world. As we move from being feeling, sensing newborns, infants, and children to losing touch with what we sense and feel, we experience our first disconnection from our body. This is when body separation or objectification begins. Dr. Niva Piran, a leading researcher in embodiment and the creator of the developmental theory of embodiment, calls this "othering."

Years ago, I heard Dr. Piran speak at a conference about her qualitative study of young girls ages nine to fourteen. Over the course of several years, she gathered stories from their lives, which helped her identify five dimensions of embodiment. Like many in the audience, I was moved to tears by accounts of girls who once felt agency and freedom in their bodies, only to lose it as they grew older. These girls reported having fun, connecting and collaborating with others without competition and comparison. They were attuned to their needs and desires, responding to them with joy—until something disrupted this capacity. The girls began to focus more on their external appearance than on their internal experience, which led to a loss of agency and autonomy. Instead of cooperating and connecting with their same-sex peers, which up until then had been natural to their female bodies, they became more focused on competition, comparison, and self-judgment. As Dr. Piran notes, when our relationship with our body is disrupted, the body becomes an uncomfortable "other."[7]

The process of "othering" creates a profound change and breeds disempowerment. We lose our sense of individual agency, becoming further detached from our bodies and our sensory experiences as we stop listening to ourselves. As a result, it becomes harder to understand and trust our bodies, making it difficult to feel safe within ourselves. I sensed that my tears, along with those of the other women, stemmed from a shared understanding. Dr. Piran's words struck a deep chord with many of us, as we have faced—and continue to face—similar challenges.

With daughters around the same age as those in Dr. Piran's study, I found myself reflecting on my own daughter. At the time, she was twelve and grappling with the changes in her body in a world that often instills fear in young girls and women regarding their natural transformations. Dr. Piran's research served as a poignant reminder of how prevalent this feeling of othering is. Women and girls are bonded through a shared suffering related to their bodies. We also have the power to heal by reconnecting with our bodies and supporting one another in this process. Beneath the disrupted relationships we have with ourselves lie our bodies, waiting to be seen, felt, and heard once again.

When My Othering Began

Take a moment to pause and notice how the above information has landed inside of you. Do you notice any emotional shift or body tension? Can you connect with the innocent little girl you were before othering began? The girl who simply belonged? Try to hold that young part of yourself with compassion and understanding. Imagine recognizing this innocent little girl in every woman you meet.

Viewing Your Body as a Relationship, Not an Image

Starting in childhood and adolescence, we often move away from the natural freedom and ease that young girls feel in their bodies and become preoccupied with how our bodies look rather than how they feel. In chapter 1 we explored why it's so easy to objectify our bodies and prioritize appearance over relationships. We live in a world that encourages disconnection from our bodies, making it easy to disengage and challenging to reconnect. Because the issue of body image—or what I call "body as image"—is so pervasive, we'll return to it throughout this book.

Body-image disturbance is real and affects every one of us. It arises from a complex mix of feelings, thoughts, memories, associations, and—most important—sensations. Sensations are often overlooked in discussions about body image, but they play a vital role. We will examine this more in depth in chapter 3, but for now it's important to recognize how focusing on the body as an image impacts your ability to form an embodied relationship with yourself.

When you see your body as just an image, you lose your chance to build a genuine relationship with it. Think about getting to know someone new: You might first be attracted to their appearance, but as time progresses you become less concerned about their looks and more interested in who they are and how you feel in their presence. You become curious about their interests, their likes and dislikes, and what makes them happy or unhappy. If you focused solely on how they looked, you would miss out on deeper intimacy. The same is true for our relationship with our bodies.

I don't expect you to stop seeing your body as an image overnight, and you shouldn't expect that of yourself either. Building a new, more embodied relationship with your body is a gradual process that you have already engaged with by reading this book. For now, simply notice that when you view your body as an image, you are participating in the othering that Dr. Piran describes—a process that distances you from true embodiment. This isn't your fault; it's the result of cultural conditioning. Learning to see your body differently is essential, but it takes time and patience to overcome this training.

One of the first steps in this process is to notice when you relate to your body in a neutral or connected way rather than through image. You might think, "That never happens to me—I am always focused on how I look!" But consider if there are times when your body image feels quiet or neutral. The following practice will help you identify and appreciate those moments, even if they're subtle or fleeting.

Moments of Embodied Connection

Think about the last time you spontaneously laughed or smiled. Choose a moment that brings a smile to your face when you recall it. It could be a moment of all-out joy or it could be something small, like laughing at your favorite show or playing with your pet.

1. Close your eyes or soften and rest your gaze. Allow the image of this moment to appear in your mind's eye.

2. How would you describe the scene? What do you see around you? Where were you? Were you alone or with a person or animal?

3. What was your body doing? Was it still? In movement? What was the movement like? Was it an action or activity?

4. As you think back to this moment, did you have any negative thoughts of your body image? I don't mean before or after, but right in that moment.

5. If not, what was present instead?

Take some time to write about this moment on a postcard or create a note in your phone. You may wish to title it "My Moment of Body Connection." Describe what brought you joy and made you smile. What was happening to allow you to shift from seeing your body as an image to being in relationship with it in the moment? Whether you realized it or not, this moment was embodied. You likely have more of these moments than you think. Use your postcard or note as a reminder that there is a different way to relate to your body—one that can soothe feelings of separation and otherness.

When Your Body Became a Problem Out in the World

Whatever impacted me, imprinted within me.
—SOFIE, STUDY PARTICIPANT

I had to release from internalizing the negative.
—JG, STUDY PARTICIPANT

How much of the cultural view was internalized?
—MAGGIE, STUDY PARTICIPANT

There was so much pain my body held from the external view of it.
—SOPHIA, STUDY PARTICIPANT

I'm working toward it all. But it doesn't come naturally.
—PEARL, STUDY PARTICIPANT

We have already established that women share the experience of living in a world that encourages disembodiment. As Jade, one of the study participants, put it, "everyone is struggling." While we share this cultural experience, each of us has had an individual journey with our body, a journey with its own unique challenges. No one is born believing that their body is a problem. This belief develops over time when we feel that our body is a burden to ourselves, to others, and to the world. The timing and circumstances that caused you to start othering your body were different for you than for your siblings or friends. Once you adopted the idea that your body is a problem, you internalized the notion that it needed to be changed or fixed. It's important to understand where and how this belief originated.

I once heard a Dharma talk by the Buddhist teacher JoAnna Hardy, who posed an intriguing question: "What has it been like for your body to be out in the world?"[8] This question sparked my curiosity and prompted me to reflect on my own body's experiences of being in this world. I noticed it was easier to answer this question from my mind, relying on familiar stories about my body rather than listening to my body itself. I listened to her talk again and realized she wasn't asking what I thought it was like for my body to exist in this world—she was inviting me to consider what I truly believed it was like *for my body*! This subtle shift in perspective calls us to a deeper, more embodied understanding of ourselves.

Your Body's Developmental Timeline in the World

Your relationship with your body is shaped by the different stages of development you move through in life. Each stage—from early childhood to adolescence and adulthood—brings unique experiences and challenges. By reflecting on your personal journey through these developmental stages, you can begin to understand how your sense of embodiment has changed over time.

Approach the following questions as a conversation with your body itself. Start by envisioning yourself sitting or walking next to your body as this dialogue unfolds. As you consider what it was like for your body at different stages of development, journal or make a recording about your sensory experience or visual memories of each time. For some age ranges, you may have both sensory and visual observations; for other age ranges one perspective may be more relevant than the other. Imagine what your body would share about its experiences during each period, working up to your current age. I have included examples of each type of reflection (sensory and visual) in the first two sections below.

As you engage in this reflection, you may notice a range of emotions arising as you listen to what your body is trying to communicate—insights that may differ from your usual understanding. Pay attention to signals that your body is at capacity and take breaks whenever needed. Approach your discoveries with a gentle mindset, as if you were encountering them for the first time. This will allow your body to receive the understanding it has always sought.

Reflect in small increments, one timeframe at a time, rather than in broad stages. Our bodies grow and change rapidly, sending different messages at each stage of development. Take your time with each period, moving gradually up to your present age.

BIRTH TO AGE FIVE: What do you imagine it was like for your body to be in the world for the first five years after you were born? Was your body seen as a problem by the world? What does your body wish to share with you about this time? What do you believe it would tell you about how it really wanted to be and be seen?

Example response:

Regarding my sensory body, I imagine it was hard for me to enter the world. I was a sensitive child, and there was a great deal happening around me at that time that felt unsafe. Because I was physically and emotionally sensitive, my body would probably have told me that people misunderstood me. I was and still am sensitive to many things, including textures, tastes, and smells. I am not difficult, just different. My body would say, "I wish I could have been seen and accepted as I am and not forced to change. I wish people didn't see me as being difficult."

AGES SIX TO TEN: What do you imagine it was like for your body to be in the world from ages six to ten? Was your body seen as a problem by the world? What does your body wish to share with you about this time? What do you believe it would tell you about how it really wanted to be and be seen?

Example response:

During these ages, my sensory body was still the same—I was very sensitive to the outside world. I became quiet to cope. My body as an image started to become a problem in the world during this time. My classmates teased me for being small and skinny. I was told I was invisible. My body would say, "I am a sensitive system. I am growing the way I am supposed to grow. I can't help the size I am. I am not invisible. I want to be seen for who I am."

AGES ELEVEN TO FOURTEEN: What do you imagine it was like for your body to be in the world from ages eleven to fourteen? Was your body seen as a problem by the world? What does your body wish to share with you about this time? What do you believe it would tell you about how it really wanted to be and be seen?

AGES FOURTEEN TO EIGHTEEN: What do you imagine it was like for your body to be in the world from ages fourteen to eighteen? Was your body seen as a problem by the world? What does your body wish to share with you about this time? What do you believe it would tell you about how it really wanted to be and be seen?

AGES EIGHTEEN TO TWENTY-ONE: What do you imagine it was like for your body to be in the world from ages eighteen to twenty-one? Was your body seen as a problem by the world? What does your body wish to share with you about this time? What do you believe it would tell you about how it really wanted to be and be seen?

AGES TWENTY-ONE TO TWENTY-FIVE: What do you imagine it was like for your body to be in the world from ages twenty-one to twenty-five? Was your body seen as a problem by the world? What does your body wish to share with you about this time? What do you believe it would tell you about how it really wanted to be and be seen?

AGES TWENTY-FIVE TO THIRTY-FIVE: What do you imagine it was like for your body to be in the world from ages twenty-five to thirty-five? Was your body seen as a problem by the world? What does your body wish to share with you about this time? What do you believe it would tell you about how it really wanted to be and be seen?

AGES THIRTY-FIVE TO FORTY-FIVE: What do you imagine it was like for your body to be in the world from ages thirty-five to forty-five?

Was your body seen as a problem by the world? What does your body wish to share with you about this time? What do you believe it would tell you about how it really wanted to be and be seen?

AGES FORTY-FIVE TO FIFTY-FIVE: What do you imagine it was like for your body to be in the world from ages forty-five to fifty-five? Was your body seen as a problem by the world? What does your body wish to share with you about this time? What do you believe it would tell you about how it really wanted to be and be seen?

AGES FIFTY-FIVE TO SIXTY-FIVE: What do you imagine it was like for your body to be in the world from ages fifty-five to sixty-five? Was your body seen as a problem by the world? What does your body wish to share with you about this time? What do you believe it would tell you about how it really wanted to be and be seen?

AGES SIXTY-FIVE TO SEVENTY-FIVE: What do you imagine it was like for your body to be in the world from ages sixty-five to seventy-five? Was your body seen as a problem by the world? What does your body wish to share with you about this time? What do you believe it would tell you about how it really wanted to be and be seen?

AGES SEVENTY-FIVE TO EIGHTY-FIVE: What do you imagine it was like for your body to be in the world from ages seventy-five to eighty-five? Was your body seen as a problem by the world? What does your body wish to share with you about this time? What do you believe it would tell you about how it really wanted to be and be seen?

AGES EIGHTY-FIVE TO PRESENT: What do you imagine it was like for your body to be in the world from ages eighty-five to the present? Was your body seen as a problem by the world? What does your body wish to share with you about this time? What do you believe it wants to tell you about how it really wanted to be and be seen?

Pause here for a moment. This exercise probably revealed to you that each stage of development comes with its unique challenges and issues. It may have brought up emotions as you realize it has not always been easy or safe for your body in this world and that women's bodies face obstacles at every stage of life. We live in a world that marginalizes and oppresses bodies, compares and criticizes them, sets high expectations, and values certain bodies while devaluing and disregarding others. This makes simply existing in this world especially difficult. Sit quietly and say the following phrases to yourself:

- *May I now understand what my body has endured out in this world, including the messages it has received, the beliefs it has held, and the judgments and shame it has experienced.*

- *May I come to understand that because of these messages, it was easy to separate from, dislike, belittle, judge, and be unkind to my body.*

- *Through this understanding, may I ignite the commitment to heal, balance, and repair this relationship. May I come to understand that I never asked for it to be this way.*

This practice is challenging! Do your best to embrace curiosity, even if the path forward doesn't feel clear in this moment. To conclude, take a moment to integrate with the following practice before moving on with your day.

When There Was Ease

This practice is available as an audio recording at www.shambhala.com/body-forgiveness-practices.

1. Close your eyes or keep them open with a soft, relaxed gaze.

2. Shift your body from side to side and begin a gentle rocking or swaying motion.

3. Feel into this rocking motion as you imagine back to a time, perhaps even before you were aware of yourself as an individual, when your body felt at ease, alive, released, unrestrained, natural, unburdened, and not a problem. This could even be a time before you were born.

4. Imagine the ability to rest within this feeling. Maybe your body continues to sway or rock, or maybe it finds its way into another physical expression, such as curling up, folding over, or even lying down. Though your mind may not believe that your body was ever at ease, your body still remembers this time, even if it was long ago. Allow your body to remember it right now.

5. Allow any images that could represent this inner feeling of ease to arise. Note this image to yourself and remember it as a shortcut back to this feeling of unburdened aliveness that is always within your body and waiting to be felt.

6. Slowly open your eyes and pause to notice even the most minor shift into ease. You may wish to journal on your experience.

As you reach the end of this chapter, take a moment to honor the courage it takes to revisit your origins and explore the many ways your relationship with your body has shifted over time. You have begun the process of meeting your body anew: moving beyond old stories of disconnection and judgment and opening to the possibility of a more compassionate, embodied relationship. This journey is not about erasing the challenges or bypassing the pain but about cultivating a deeper understanding of how you have arrived at this moment and how your body has always been present, waiting for you to listen. Each reflection and practice you've engaged in is a step toward healing the separation and rediscovering the inherent wisdom and kindness within your body.

In the next chapter, we will delve even deeper into this reconnection by exploring the sensory body—the foundation of your embodied experience. We'll look closely at the ways your senses, especially the sense of touch, shape your relationship with yourself and the world around you. By learning to listen to and trust your body's sensory signals, you'll begin to reclaim the natural communication and self-awareness that have always been your birthright.

3

UNDERSTANDING YOUR SENSORY BODY

Let the breath energy sit near places that might be tight or painful. And notice if different sensations, odors, or colors are there. No pushing, no pulling, simply being near, listening, like a good friend.[1]

—MARISELA B. GOMEZ

THE THIRD STAGE of body forgiveness is about understanding sensation and discovering your unique sensory body. In this chapter you'll be introduced to the sensory body and begin to explore what it truly means to build a real, authentic relationship with your body. This shift will enable you to experience your body in an entirely new way. The philosopher Merleau-Ponty describes the sensing body as the breathing body that experiences and inhabits the world.[2] To fully engage with the world, we need to move beyond seeing our bodies as mere objects or collections of parts and instead embrace the living, subjective experience of being in and with our body. This means viewing your body as an interconnected whole, both within yourself and with others. The journey begins with developing a deeper sense of feeling and awareness from within.

Starting with Sensations

I had to feel head-to-foot connected.
—MAGGIE, STUDY PARTICIPANT

I had to make sense of sensations.
—MEG, STUDY PARTICIPANT

Sensations are the primary way your body communicates its needs to you and to others in the world. Sensations can be seen as expressions of your body's needs, wishes, and desires. Unfortunately, as women, we are often conditioned from a young age to shift our focus and attention away from our sensory and emotional needs, our wishes and desires, and instead attend to the needs of others. Whether we choose to embrace socially constructed gender roles or hormonally driven norms of caretaking and nurturing, it is often natural for women to give to and care for others. There is nothing inherently wrong with this tendency, though it becomes problematic when it feels distressing or uncomfortable on the inside.

We often overlook the subtle sensory changes that occur each time we step aside or give up our physical or emotional needs for someone else's. If you pay close attention during these moments, you may notice a shift within your body, such as a tightness or slight contraction somewhere in your body or mind. It could be a tightening sensation in your chest, stomach, neck, back, or another area. A part of you may be quietly expressing, "I'd rather not." These moments of contraction represent tiny instances of bodily discomfort, and they can accumulate into larger feelings of stress, distress, and even illness. Learning to identify with the physical sensations associated with this contraction is an important step.

What Does Body Contraction Feel Like?

This practice will help you recognize when you are distancing yourself from what you or your body needs. To begin, let's explore some common areas in your body where you might experience contraction, so you can better understand what that sensation feels like.

1. Clench your jaw, pressing and holding your teeth together. Notice the contraction in your jaw and neck muscles. Release and repeat a few times. Focus on the difference between how the contraction feels and how the release feels. Write down a few words to describe the difference.

2. Let your head tilt slightly back and press the tip of your tongue to the roof of your mouth and hold. Notice the contraction that builds in your neck and especially your throat. Release and repeat a few times. Focus on the difference between how the contraction feels and how the release feels in your neck and throat. Write down a few words to describe the difference.

3. Take opposite hands to opposite arms, allowing your shoulders to roll inward. Squeeze your torso tightly. Notice the contraction that builds in your upper back, shoulders, and chest. Release and repeat a few times. Focus on the difference between how the contraction feels and how the release feels in your upper back, shoulders, and chest. Write down a few words to describe the difference.

4. Squeeze your naval toward the back of your body, like you are sucking in your stomach, and hold. Notice the contraction that builds very quickly in your abdominal area and back. Release and repeat a few times. Focus on the difference between how the contraction feels and how the release

feels in your stomach and back. Write down a few words to describe the difference.

5. Squeeze your hands together and hold them tightly. Notice the contraction that builds in your hands and up your arms. Release and repeat a few times. Focus on the difference between how the contraction feels and how the release feels in your hands and arms. Write down a few words to describe the difference.

6. Press your right foot firmly into the ground and notice the contraction that builds in the foot, ankle, and leg. Release and repeat a few times. Focus on the difference between how the contraction feels and how the release feels in your foot, ankle, and leg. Write down a few words to describe the difference.

7. Repeat number six on the left side.

When you finish, take a moment to journal or make an audio recording about the differences between the sensations of contraction and release. Be as detailed as you can in your observations. Becoming familiar with how contraction feels in your body can help you maintain connection with yourself when you are relating to others. When you feel a moment of contraction, that is an opportunity to pause and ask yourself, *Do I have a need that I'm ignoring? Did I just prioritize someone else's needs over my own?*

A New Definition of Pleasure

In a study I conducted on the role of self-compassion in women's recovery from disordered eating, I found that every woman I interviewed described, in her own way, the complex relationship between her needs and her experience of pleasure. Those who ignored their emotional and sensory needs often struggled to embrace pleasure in their lives.

The word *pleasure* is particularly evocative in our society, especially when it comes to female bodies. It's a loaded term, often narrowly associated with sexual experiences and orgasm. As we move forward, I invite you to embrace a broader understanding of this word. What if we viewed pleasure as any sensation that *brings comfort* to your body?

As you may have noticed in the previous practice, when we tense our bodies, we often create moments of physical discomfort that can lead us to deny, withhold, or move away from what our bodies truly need. This response can make it harder to connect with our internal sensory experiences and to recognize what release and comfort feel like. Recognizing what is comforting is one of the essential foundations for developing a new understanding and relationship with pleasure.

Pleasure is a natural state of our bodies. Our earliest experiences of pleasure are rooted in comfort. Think about how a baby seeks out soft materials, soothing sounds, gentle voices, and nurturing touch. At its core, your body still craves these same comforts today.

EMBODIED PRACTICE

Discovering Comfort in Your Body

Gather a blanket and several pillows for this practice, then take a seat in a comfortable chair.

1. Close your eyes or keep them open with a soft, relaxed gaze.

2. Inhale for a count of four and exhale for a count of four. Repeat this equalizing breath a few times.

3. Place one or two pillows behind your back and one under your feet. Place a blanket either behind your head or draped over your body. Lean into the pillow behind you, sensing the softness of its support up against your spine. Feel your feet press into the pillow on the floor. Begin to gently rock, pressing your feet and your back body into the softness of the pillows. Adjust the pillows and blanket in any way you wish if it helps to bring even 5 or 10 percent more comfort to your body in this moment.

4. Once you have found the most comfortable spot you can right now, pause and stay there for a few minutes.

5. Repeat these words either silently to yourself or out loud: *This is comfort. This is what comfort feels like inside. Comfort is pleasure.*

Practice this as often as possible to enhance your awareness of what comfort in your body feels like and to develop a new understanding of pleasure. Throughout the day, take the time to recognize when your body is comfortable and when it is not. This awareness is a crucial first step in rebuilding your relationship with pleasure and recognizing your needs.

What If Food Could Be Comforting?

In chapter 2 you explored how food can be a nurturing experience. Even if that doesn't feel true for you right now, I invite you to take a breath and stay open to discovering something new. For many of us, food no longer feels nurturing, calming, and soothing. But the bond between food and your body has deep roots that are often overlooked. Before you were born or could think about it, food was your body's first and most steadfast companion. Its role was to provide consistent support and nourishment for your body.

At birth your relationship with food shifted from automatic nourishment in the womb to relying on caregivers to meet your needs and help you develop a new relationship with food. Some of us received consistent, reliable care, while others experienced inconsistency—sometimes due to a caregiver's limitation, sometimes because of food scarcity. Even if your experiences with food were unpredictable, your body still remembers the steady nourishment it received in the womb. This memory lives on within you, and your body recalls a sense of comfort and ease.

Remembering the Comfort of Food

This reflection focuses on recalling your earliest memories of food. You may have answers based on what your caregivers or others have told you, but if there are questions you can't answer, imagine what those experiences might have been like for you. These reflections are meant to spark curiosity and a sense of wonder about your body; don't worry about knowing the right answers.

- Did you feel nurtured with food in a consistent, reliable, and predictable way? If not, what was your experience?

- Did you enjoy being fed? Did you like longer or shorter feedings? Did your body need to eat frequently or infrequently?

- Did you enjoy the calming comfort of sucking? Were you allowed to use a pacifier or suck your thumb?

- Can you recall the first food you remember enjoying? What was it? What about it brought you joy and/or comfort, perhaps even as you think about it now?

- Is this food in your life now? If yes, is your relationship with it a natural, embodied, gentle, nurturing, nonharming experience? If not, can you imagine this food ever returning to a gentle, nurturing experience?

Your body remembers how it once received nourishment. Your body and organs still prefer to receive food in a manner that feels nurturing. Consider gently rocking or swaying while you eat. This can create space to connect with your food on a sensory level, allowing you to experience it as your body once remembered.

Relearning the Language of Sensation

Sensations, which range from the obvious to the subtle, are your body's way of communicating with you in the moment. Simply put, sensation is anything you perceive through your senses—touch, sight, sound, smell, and taste. These external sensations are often easy to notice: the feel of your chair, a sound in the room, the smells in the air. But there are also internal sensations like tight muscles, achy joints, or pain. Interoception, or interoceptive awareness, is the ability to notice signals from your internal body. These can be more challenging to detect, but the good news is you can train yourself to become aware of them.

Internal sensations are often subtle—like the feeling of tension before it becomes pain, the first signs of hunger or fullness, or when you start to feel tired. Even more subtle are the signals from your organs and inner body. While it may feel strange to focus on these internal cues, they are a natural and consistent part of your body's communication. Learning to listen to and understand these signals is essential for building a relationship with your body, and it's a skill that you can develop.

One of my mentors, Dr. Cynthia Price—a leading researcher in interoceptive awareness and creator of the Mindful Awareness in Body-Oriented Therapy (MABT) program, in which I am certified—discusses how the development of interoceptive awareness is a powerful skill that can help you transition from disconnection to deeper body awareness.[3] However, it can be challenging at first.

Although we are born with the ability to listen and respond to our interoceptive signals, they often fade into the background when our thinking mind takes over—especially when we prioritize others' needs, worry, or focus on body image. Even clear signals can be drowned out when our mind dominates our attention. Body forgiveness is about relearning this natural communication with your sensory system. It requires prioritizing what you sense and feel in your body over what you think you sense and feel. This can be difficult, especially if you have spent much of your life favoring mental experiences over physical ones. Like many women, you may notice that a busy, judgmental, or worried mind often pulls you away from truly being in tune with your body.

Two Ways to Quiet the Mind

Part of the reason it's difficult to attend to our sensory experience is that our minds are constantly active and rarely still. In today's world distraction is at an all-time high, and we've been trained to focus on what we see rather than what we sense and feel. Unless we intentionally retrain our minds through practices like mindfulness and meditation—which help calm our thoughts and enhance our attention—our minds will naturally be filled with swirling activity. To counter this, we need to establish specific supports, or pillars, that help quiet the mind and make space for sensory awareness.

FIRST PILLAR: PAUSING

Pausing quiets the mind and creates space to tune in, helping you establish a new relationship with your sensations. The Buddhist meditation teacher Tara Brach describes the power of the pause as a sacred act that aligns with our body's natural rhythms and the flow of life.[4] The more you practice pausing, the more attuned you become to what is most natural for your body. Your body needs time and space to register what is happening internally. It is better to pause rather than bypass sensations or get entangled in your thoughts. When you move too quickly—physically or mentally—you can easily overlook your body's sensory signals. Even obvious sensations like pain can be missed or dismissed when you rush through life. Pausing gives you just enough time to slow down and notice what is happening in the present moment. Pausing is different from stillness; it's more like a gentle middle ground between movement and stillness. Let's practice discovering your pause.

Embodying a Moment of Pause

In chapter 2 we explored rediscovering the kind of movement you enjoyed as a child—or perhaps even in the womb. Did you do a rocking, swaying, or stretching motion? Return to that movement now or choose a movement that feels good in this moment.

1. Sit or lie down and allow your body to move gently with whatever motion you have chosen. See if you can find a few words to describe what this motion feels like inside. Is it gentle, fluid, easeful, free, calming, strong? Choose your own words.

2. With your next breath, slow the motion so you are nearly still and just notice. This almost still place is the embodied pause.

3. Move again and then slow down again. Repeat this moving and pausing rhythm a few times.

4. The next time you pause, sense what you notice. Does the pause create a noticeable internal difference? Perhaps it is an obvious body sensation, thought, or emotion. Perhaps it is new.

Practice your embodied pause several times a day to get a sense of what it feels like to slow down in both body and mind. Each time you pause and notice, you strengthen your ability to be present with your body. This presence helps you stay attuned to what you sense and feel, so that you do not let thoughts—especially critical ones—cloud your experience. Pausing is how we begin to separate sensation from thought and start to truly understand our body's communication. It also quiets external distractions, making it easier to hear what your body is telling you. As is true in building any relationship, if we're distracted or rushing, we miss the chance to connect more deeply. As you practice slowing down and pausing, you enhance your awareness and sensory understanding—an essential skill for reconnecting with your body.

SECOND PILLAR: SLOWING DOWN

The second pillar, slowing down, anchors us in noticing what's happening inside. We are enculturated to move fast, do more, and be more, and we expect our bodies to keep up with this fast pace. As a result, slowing down can be challenging. In the previous practice, Embodying a Moment of Pause, you started to experience slowing down. Unlike complete stillness—which is not accessible to most people—intentionally slowing down is more manageable. Developing this skill begins with becoming aware of how quickly we move through daily life. By consciously reducing our pace, we create space to notice present sensations and access the insights our bodies offer. As you practice slowing down and paying attention to your body, you may find that your body actually prefers a gentler, slower pace than what you currently demand of it.

The Way I Move

This reflection is meant to help you slow down and shift your focus and attention to the daily tasks you may already be doing in your body.

IN THE MORNING: As you awaken and your body emerges into the day, notice how quickly you move from lying down to getting out of bed. Do you allow your body to awaken slowly? Your body has been at rest for many hours. Do you consider how your body may wish to start the day?

Ask: *At this moment, what might my body be telling me?*

IN THE AFTERNOON: As your body rhythms wax and wane, consider how you walk from place to place. Do you shift your pace according to the natural shifts in energy that your body experiences, or do you move at the same pace throughout the day? Do you ever consider how your body may wish to move throughout the day?

Ask: *At this moment, what might my body be telling me?*

IN THE EVENING: As your day winds down and your body's energy slows down in preparation for rest, notice if your pace matches this. How are you moving your body as the natural tide of the day has shifted? Do you slow your pace as the evening comes? Do you ever consider how your body may wish to move at the end of the day?

Ask: *At this moment, what might my body be telling me?*

This reflection will help you become aware of and curious about how you move your body throughout the day and, more important, whether it matches the nature of your body's natural pace and rhythm.

Body Agency and the Importance of Building Sensory Knowledge

Neuroscience has shown that the more connected we are to our sensory experience, the better we can soothe and regulate emotions and thoughts and the greater sense of agency we feel in our body. Agency means feeling capable in your body, and developing a sense of agency is crucial to building a healthier relationship with yourself.

No matter your abilities or level of functioning, everybody (and every body) has the potential to cultivate agency. It is important to understand that agency isn't defined by society's standards of what a body can or cannot do—it's about staying connected to what your body is naturally capable of. When we feel disembodied we lose trust in our body's capabilities and its value, both in the world and in our own healing. Unless you are familiar with somatic psychotherapy, it's rare to walk into a therapist's office and say, "Can you help me get in touch with my sensations so I can reconnect with my body and sense of agency?" Yet that's exactly what heightened interoceptive awareness can offer: the capacity to regain agency, build inner safety, and foster a new appreciation for your body. The following reflection will help you become more aware of your sensing body.

EMBODIED PRACTICE

Sensing a Moment

1. I invite you to touch your hands together, palm to palm, and notice the temperature of your skin. Are your hands warm, cool, hot, cold? Do they feel hard, soft, smooth, or rough? Now press your palms together and stop at the amount of pressure that feels pleasant. How do you know it is pleasing to you? What happens inside as you feel this amount of pressure?

2. Release the touch and look around your space. Allow your eyes to land on the most colorful object in your space. What do you see? What happens inside as you see this color? Does the color evoke a shift within you somehow? Is it a pleasant color? If so, how do you know it is pleasing to you? Is it unpleasant? If so, how do you know it's unpleasant to you?

3. Notice if you can hear any sounds, whether close by or far away. Is the sound pleasant or unpleasant? How do you know? What happens inside when you hear or even imagine this sound?

4. Take notice of any pleasant smells around you. If nothing stands out, imagine a scent that is pleasing to you. What do you enjoy about this scent? What happens inside when you smell or imagine it?

5. Recall a flavor or taste you find pleasing. What do you enjoy about this taste? How do you know you enjoy this taste? What happens inside when you imagine this taste?

You may already be familiar with practices like this, especially if you have participated in mindfulness training, which often begins with the first foundation of mindfulness: exploring body sensations and breath. This practice adds a unique dimension by encouraging you to ask: *What happens inside?* This question is about interoception—our ability to sense internal bodily states. While external sensations are often easy to notice, they also produce internal experiences that we may overlook because we have become conditioned to turn away from them. Asking what happens inside shifts your attention from simply acknowledging a sensation to being curious about how it feels internally.

When you ignore your body's internal messages your thoughts tend to take over. Evolutionary theory suggests that humans are wired for self-protection to seek out what feels pleasant and avoid what feels unpleasant. When we experience sensations that are particularly pleasant or unpleasant, they create a lasting impact on our minds. As we dwell in our thoughts on these sensations, we unconsciously distance ourselves from actually sensing them in the body.

While we're caught up in our thoughts, many changes are happening within our interoceptive body, often outside our awareness. Each sensory experience leaves us with feelings that go beyond just our thoughts. The question *What's happening inside?* becomes a crucial anchor, redirecting your focus back to your inner experience instead of letting your mind spiral into endless thought.

Anchoring Back Inside

Your sensations can serve as anchors, helping you feel more grounded throughout the day. Many daily rituals you already practice can be transformed into sensory-aware moments. For example, I love warmth: warm showers, tea, blankets, and sunlight. When I drink my morning cup of tea, I don't just savor the taste. I also feel the warmth of the cup in my hands and the soothing sensation spreading through my body. On one level, my mind registers enjoyment, but if I practice pausing and slowing down, my mind quiets and I become aware of what's happening inside. I recognize that there is a *quality* about the warmth in my body as the tea travels from my mouth down through my throat, into my chest, and finally reaches my stomach, producing a soothing and calming effect inside me. It's not just heat—it's a comforting sensation. My mind appreciates this ritual, and so does my entire sensory system. Now, whenever I have my cup of tea, I remind myself: *At this moment, I am soothing and calming my body.*

Sensory-Aware Moments

What do you currently know about your sensing body? Consider what helps you anchor yourself and return to the present. This reflection invites you to explore your senses more deeply by asking: What's happening *inside*?

- In chapter 2 we explored your relationship with touch. What do you notice about how you experience touch? Are there types of touch you find appealing? Are there certain areas of your body where touch feels especially pleasant, unpleasant, or neutral? How do you recognize these sensations, and what happens inside when you feel them?

- What is your relationship with sound? Are there sounds you find appealing, unpleasant, or neutral? How do you sense the difference? What happens inside in those moments?

- Do you prefer quiet, solitude, and calm spaces, or are you someone who enjoys lively environments and being around others? How do you know when you feel too alone or too crowded? What happens inside in those moments?

- How do you respond to different textures, such as the feel of clothing on your skin? Which textures do you enjoy and which ones feel unpleasant or neutral? How do you sense these preferences, and what happens inside when you notice them?

- What is your relationship to the texture of food? Are there certain textures of food you find more pleasant, unpleasant, or neutral? How do you recognize your response to these textures, and what happens inside when you notice them?

Awareness of sensory sensitivities often goes back to childhood. For example, when I reflect on my own experience, I remember preferring soft, fluid fabrics and disliking tight or binding clothing. I never liked the feeling of socks slipping down my legs or feet, and I still have the same sensitivities today. When I observe what happens on the inside, I notice that tight clothing makes my breath become shallow and pulls my focus away from my body's sensations and increases preoccupying thoughts—often about body image. The discomfort disrupts my thoughts, but recognizing this allows me to anchor myself and make adjustments to support my body's comfort.

These are just a few examples of sensory sensitivity you might explore. Even if you are unaware of any sensations or sensitivities, it's still valuable to ask the question. Doing so draws your attention to your body and helps you develop the ability to name and identify sensory experiences. Dr. Price calls this "body literacy," and it's the first step in awakening the connection between your sensory system and your brain.

Sensations as Messages, Not Complaints

When we intentionally or unintentionally ignore our body's signals, our ability to recognize them gradually declines. Over time, some cues may fade while others become more pronounced. Take hunger cues, for example. Many women say, "I don't eat breakfast because I'm not hungry in the morning." Yet your stomach typically empties within two to five hours, depending on the size of your last meal. If you've been asleep for more than five hours and your last meal was even earlier than that, your stomach is likely empty. If you don't feel hungry, it's often because your body's subtle and obvious signals have been ignored for too long. If these signals go unheeded, your body may eventually stop sending them—or it may send louder messages instead, such as intense sensation or pain.

One of my participants, Meg, said, "I kept dismissing my body's signals as complaints instead of seeing them as messages." You may also find yourself viewing your body's sensations as nothing more than complaints. When we overlook subtle, interoceptive cues, sensations often get louder. As they escalate, they can become more intimidating. Think about what it feels like when someone yells at you for no apparent reason. That's like the experience we have when our interoceptive signals grow louder and we still don't understand how to listen. We may find them annoying or misinterpret them as distress signals.

Instead of dismissing or feeling distressed about these signals, try pausing and slowing down. Remind yourself, *Oh yes, this is my body's way of communicating with me.* This reminder can help you reconnect with the truth of your body's messages. Your body is simply trying to talk to you, and interoception is its language.

EMBODIED PRACTICE

Sensing What's Here Now

This practice is available as an audio recording at www.shambhala.com/body-forgiveness-practices. It is designed to help you connect with your body's signals by focusing on an area that commonly holds tension. In my experience teaching therapeutic yoga, the neck and jaw are frequent sites of tension for many people. For now, I encourage you to concentrate on this area. In later chapters you'll have the opportunity to explore other areas on your own. You may want to use a pillow to support your arms during this practice. Feel free to close your eyes or maintain a soft, relaxed gaze.

1. Take a comfortable seat and begin with a deep inhale followed by a long exhale to release tension.

2. Place a pillow underneath your elbows to support your arms and bring a hand to either side of your neck.

3. Gently move your fingers up and down the large muscles of your neck, noticing any areas that stand out. Describe what you feel. Is it tense, tight, lumpy, stuck, stiff, congested, bumpy, or something else? If you find a spot like this, pause and let your fingertips rest there for a few breaths.

4. As you stay with this area, continue to describe what you notice, using any words that come to mind.

5. Next, move your fingertips up to your jaw and trace along your jawline from the center to the back, just beneath your ears. Glide your fingers from center to back and back to center a few times, noticing any sensations. Do you find areas that feel tender, achy, sore, or tense? If so, pause and let your fingertips rest there for a few breaths.

6. While you linger here, continue to describe what you notice, using whatever words feel right.

7. Release your hands and take a deep breath. Recall which sensation stood out most, where it was located, and the words you used to describe it.

8. Gently move your neck side to side and open and close your jaw a few times. Check in with the area you focused on and notice if the sensation has changed.

You may want to write down your observations. I encourage you to repeat these steps daily to enhance your body awareness. By focusing on discovering, noticing, and describing areas of tension, you strengthen your internal communication system. Each time you do this, you create a greater sense of safety and protection within your body and mind. In chapter 4 you will learn why establishing this sense of safety is so important. Your body appreciates the time you take to notice, care for, and approach it in new and gentle ways.

Getting to Know Your Internal Body

Our current medical system often relies on the biomedical model, which tends to view humans as a collection of biological parts. To be clear, I value Western medical knowledge and rely on it extensively. I also recognize that not all medical professionals strictly adhere to this model, and I've been fortunate to receive care from many who do not. Still, much of the training remains rooted in a reductionist and materialist perspective, which can reinforce the idea that we know little about our own bodies—especially our internal experiences and what might be right for us.

Consider what it would be like to connect with your internal body in a way that helps you understand how you're feeling and what you need. This connection can help you communicate more clearly with your healthcare providers and may even allow you to recognize your body's needs before anyone else does.

You have the ability to sense and understand your internal body long before anyone else can tell you about it. By retraining yourself to notice sensory information, you can question, discern, and respond to what is best for your body. Imagine having the internal wisdom to know which foods are right for you rather than depending on the latest trends in diet culture. You can also learn to discern daily needs, such as how much rest, movement, or social connection you require. The more you develop your sensory awareness, the better you can communicate your body's needs. Picture going into an appointment equipped with the language of your body: "I feel discomfort on my right side," or "The pain is located internally here, not there."

Getting to know your internal body enhances your sense of agency and ultimately improves the care you receive. To deepen this connection with your body, it's essential to understand it in a more embodied way.

A Unique Body Scan for Embodying Your Internal Body

This practice is available as an audio recording at www.shambhala.com/body-forgiveness-practices. Let's explore your internal body in a new way, focusing on your organs to foster discovery and respect. This body scan invites you to move gently and use your imagination to connect with different areas of your body. The italicized words serve as a *body mantra*, a repetitive phrase you can use during practice and anytime you want to connect and be present with your internal body.

This is a longer body scan, so I encourage you to move slowly, focusing on one area at a time. You can begin by sitting, lying down, or standing, and feel free to change your position as needed.

1. Begin by taking a deep inhale and a big exhale. Place one hand on your head and one behind your neck. Slowly move your head from side to side and front to back, imagining you are embracing your brain and nervous system. Your brain is the compassionate master of your body, constantly receiving and sending information to every region and organ. It works tirelessly to maintain your body's communication and balance. This is the power station of all your sense organs and sensations—it is where your body's interconnectedness happens. Your central nervous system communicates your wish to move, responding instantly to your intentions, many hundreds of times a day. Think about the hundreds of movements you make every day.

2. Take a deep breath, then gently round your spine back and straighten it forward. Place one hand on your chest and one somewhere on your back where it's easy to reach so you

can feel your spine move. Imagine the spaces between each vertebrae opening and closing as you move, massaging the discs in between and awakening the forty-three pairs of spinal nerves in your peripheral nervous system. You are awakening your sensory and autonomic nervous system, where all sensations and feelings of safety are born.

3. Pause and reflect on your brain, the sophisticated master communicator within you, the quiet ruler and connector of all.

Here is my center of higher consciousness and knowledge.

4. Take another deep breath and place your hands on your heart. With each inhale open your arms wide, and on the exhale return your hands to your heart. Your heart is the power center of your body, pumping over two thousand gallons of nourishing blood to your organs, muscles, and extremities every day, generating your internal life force. It also feels deeply, sensing the world through your autonomic nervous system. It knows when you feel safe and connected and when you feel unsafe and disconnected.

5. Pause with your hands on your heart and sense its beating. Imagine your blood energizing you and transmitting your life force.

Here is where my most profound wisdom and highest self reside.

6. Place your hands on your ribs. As you inhale, gently lift your ribs, and as you exhale, let them soften. Imagine embracing your lungs, the other half of your body's power center. Your lungs and heart rely on each other. Your heart relies on your lungs' ability to properly clean and oxygenate your blood.

With each inhale, your diaphragm helps your lungs fill with oxygen, and each exhale releases carbon dioxide. The heart and the lungs work together seamlessly, circulating blood through your body in about sixteen seconds without you having to think about it.

7. Pause with your hands on either side of your ribcage, holding your heart and lungs, sensing their rhythmic dance with each breath.

Here, with each breath I take, I receive. With each breath I release, I let go. Here, I am connected to my life force. I am alive; I am alive.

8. Inhale and exhale, wrapping your arms around your stomach, or embrace a pillow in this area. Gently rock back and forth rhythmically and imagine this area as the container of all that nourishes you. Your stomach digests and absorbs nutrients and fluids, moving in rhythmic waves to transfer nutrients to your small intestine. Because of its relationship with your autonomic nervous system, your stomach is also a sensitive, feeling organ that registers feelings of fear as well as safety and calm, which is its preferred state for proper digestion.

9. Pause your rocking and hold your stomach.

Here lives my emotional self, my sensitive soul.

10. Inhale and exhale, placing a hand or pillow on the upper right quadrant of your belly beneath your ribcage. Press your feet into the ground, imagining the steady, solid presence of your liver. Your liver is your largest solid organ and plays a vital role in nearly every organ system in your body. It cleanses and detoxifies your blood and helps maintain chemical homeostasis throughout your body. It has the most

extraordinary regenerative capacity of any organ and, if unwell, will work its hardest to heal and regenerate itself.

11. Pause and hold your liver, honoring its capacity.

Here lives my groundedness and my life's direction.

12. Inhale and exhale, placing a hand or pillow across your belly and another across your mid- to lower back. Breathe into this space where your pancreas lives, embracing this organ of regulation and metabolic energy. Considered both an organ and a gland, the pancreas releases essential digestive enzymes and produces insulin, helping you regulate your energy and blood-sugar levels. It also supports your other vital organs, such as your liver, kidneys, heart, and brain.

13. Pause to consider your pancreas as a caregiver for your other organs.

Here lives my happiness, my gratitude, and stepping into my life.

14. Inhale and exhale, placing your hands or a pillow across your back just below your rib cage. Gently lean side to side and bend forward and backward, awakening your kidneys, your body's powerful filters and regulators. Your kidneys maintain homeostasis in your body by filtering your blood, maintaining proper electrolyte balance, and regulating your blood pressure. They have a unique bond with the heart, constantly communicating to keep you safe, stable, and alive.

15. Pause to honor the giver of balance, life, and calming energy.

Here, may I live unafraid. May I know peace.

This practice is a reminder of your body's interconnectedness. Each organ relies on the others for support, working together to maintain balance and repair. The cycle of belonging and mutual need is always at work as your body strives to regulate and repair itself.

I hope this practice inspires deeper appreciation and wonderment for your internal body. Use it anytime to view your body differently, especially during challenging body-image moments to reconnect with a more spiritual and compassionate understanding of your internal body.

This chapter is just the beginning of recognizing and developing your internal communication system. From here, you'll learn to strengthen this powerful connection with your body. For now, I encourage you to keep practicing pausing and slowing down. With each breath and step, your body is communicating with you.

> There is deep wisdom within our very flesh, if we can only come to our senses and feel it.
>
> **—WIDELY ATTRIBUTED TO ELIZABETH A. BEHNKE**

4

UNDERSTANDING YOUR BODY'S INTERNAL STORY

Whether you are working through deep fear and shame or a less acute emotional reaction, your inner freedom will arise from bringing attention to how the experience is expressed in your body.[1]

—TARA BRACH

My body didn't create any offense. It just needed understanding.

—JOSEPHINE, STUDY PARTICIPANT

THE FOURTH STAGE of body forgiveness is about developing a new understanding of how your unique life experiences have manifested within your body. By exploring these experiences and their significance, you can discover new ways to relate to and address them. Now that you've seen how external messages can disrupt your internal view, it's time to gently investigate how internalized messages and personal experiences have shaped your body's experience. Let's begin by exploring the embodied experience of your body's center.

Finding Your Center

In yoga each asana, or pose, develops from your body's midline. Here we'll use a variation of *Dandasana* (Staff Pose) to help you connect with your midline and find your center.

1. Sit on the floor with your knees bent and your back supported by a large pillow between you and the wall. If it is uncomfortable for you to get up and down from the floor, you can sit in a chair with a pillow behind you.

2. Place your arms alongside your body, fingertips touching the ground or chair.

3. Slowly straighten one leg at a time, pressing your back into the pillow. Bend and straighten your legs until both are straight. Repeat a few times.

4. Pause and notice the sensations in the front and back of your body. Imagine a string gently lifting you from your navel up through your chest and throat. Move your body up and down as if this invisible string is lifting you.

5. Where do you sense your center—in the front, back, or both? Can you feel it along your spine or from your navel to your chest? Maybe you feel it in more than one place.

6. Describe what your center feels like using words such as supported, held, strong, open, tired, alive, or able to breathe.

Descriptive words reflect internal experiences, not physical appearance. This is important since, due to cultural conditioning, many women feel particularly dissatisfied with this area of their body and disconnected from their midline and the strength there.

If body-image issues interrupt your exploration, pause and remind yourself, *This is a moment of disembodiment.* Gently sway or rock to reconnect and allow yourself to learn something new.

Practice daily until finding your center becomes second nature—whether seated, walking, or lying down. This awareness means the practice is becoming embodied. Recognizing when you feel centered will also help you notice when you're out of balance or disconnected.

A New Embodied Way to Understand Triggers

You may know the term *triggered,* which often refers to being set off emotionally. The problem is that when we acknowledge being triggered, it draws attention to thoughts rather than what's happening in our bodies. You've practiced identifying your body's center; triggering events can push you off that center, leading to feelings of unsafety and unease. By noticing these sensations and staying with them, you help your body return to balance. Instead of saying "I'm triggered," try "I'm away from my middle" or "That throws me off my center." These phrases help reconnect you with your body and rediscover what it feels like to return to your center.

Many experiences can push us off-center, making it challenging to maintain a sense of internal connection and embodiment. Without understanding how our bodies have absorbed these experiences, we may see our bodies as enemies. As Josephine, a study participant, said, "There was all the stuff in the outside world I had to make sense of, and then there were the exceptional experiences that impacted my body. I had to make sense of those too."

The Impact of Exceptional Experiences

What was imprinted, impacted! It is still in my body
as a default protection.
—SOFIE, STUDY PARTICIPANT

We are wired to seek safety and avoid danger. Uncomfortable and alarming sensations are our body's way of communicating, but they can create unease as our mind tries to understand and interpret them in an effort to protect us. You might know the story of an exceptional experience and think you've resolved it, yet you still feel disconnected from your body or unclear inside. Even when we understand an experience intellectually, our bodies may still feel discomfort or disconnection. Making sense in the mind alone doesn't address the body's experience. Even years later, your body can feel off-center and perceive your surroundings as unsafe.

We all have unique life stories shaped by our families and ancestors. Some experiences feel safe and natural, while others do not. Events that throw us off balance are often traumatic—they feel unnatural and were never meant to occur. I call these "exceptional experiences"—distinct responses, unique to each of us, that leave us feeling unsafe in our bodies and the world. For example, like me, many of you are likely the adult child of a caregiver or parent who struggled with addiction. However, my body's response to that experience is different from yours. Our body's individuality makes our experiences exceptional, even within similar stories.

Everyone encounters exceptional experiences. In *The Body Keeps the Score*, trauma expert Bessel van der Kolk notes that these experiences can reorganize our internal reality and affect the "core of who we are," especially how we perceive events and what happens in our bodies.[2] "The body keeps the score" has become a widely used phrase to describe the impact of trauma on the body. However, instead of saying "your body keeps the score," I prefer to say "your body knows the truth." Your body senses and feels events immediately, often before your mind has the chance to interpret or understand them. Even if your mind can't fully understand or remember, your body holds valuable insights into these experiences and has been waiting for you to recognize it.

Exceptional experiences shape your life by how they affect your body. Many of us live disconnected from our body's messages and thus feel unsafe and confused. When we can't make sense of what we feel, sensations get louder and more frightening. You may try to think your way out, but focusing on stories and thoughts moves us away from sensing what's going on inside when we have these memories or thoughts. Instead, trust that your body retains the thoughts and feelings of past experiences through sensations. Reconnecting with these sensations will help you make sense of what your body remembers.

EMBODIED PRACTICE

Your Body as a Canvas

PART ONE: DISCOVERING BODY LOCATION

Through creativity and imagination, this practice helps you identify where exceptional experiences reside in your body.

1. Imagine your body as a blank canvas.

2. Think of an exceptional experience that stands out for you. Instead of telling the story about it, where would you paint it on your body? Is the paint on the surface or would you paint it deeper inside as well? Let your answer be spontaneous—don't give it much thought.

3. Think of another exceptional experience and imagine where you would paint it on your body. Repeat this several more

times. Notice if you return repeatedly to certain areas of your body and if one stands out.

4. What drew you to this area? Focus on sensory details—tension, knots, aches, or pain.

5. Place a hand on the area and say the words your body longs to hear: *I sense you and I feel you.*

This practice is the first step in identifying where you've felt exceptional experiences in your body. For example, after losing a parent early, I remember feeling a tightness and nausea in my stomach. Even now, grief settles in my stomach. I encourage you to explore whether the areas in your body that held these feelings in the past still feel alive now.

Returning to Your Center of Safety and Ease

In 1994 the neuroscientist, psychologist, and researcher Dr. Stephen Porges introduced polyvagal theory, which transformed our understanding of the autonomic nervous system—the body's safety and regulation center—by highlighting the crucial role of the vagus nerve.[3] The theory explains that the vagus nerve is central to how our bodies respond to stress, safety, and connection. It plays a crucial role in influencing our behavior and overall health by helping restore our organs to a safe state and maintaining our body's balance, or homeostasis, by continuously registering sensory information and facilitating automatic communication between the body and brain. In essence, the vagus nerve acts as an internal surveillance system, constantly monitoring for cues of safety and danger.

Dr. Porges coined the term *neuroception* to describe the body's ability to detect and interpret what is happening internally from the environment and from interaction with others at a sensory level.

Consider a frightening event or sensation. Whether you're aware of it, your energy shifts into a state of arousal (sympathetic activation of the autonomic nervous system). Your body releases stress hormones like adrenaline and cortisol to help mobilize your energy and to prepare you to fight, flee, or freeze. During sympathetic activation, it's common to experience an increased heart rate, anxiety, a sense of muscular tightness in your body, and a mind preoccupied with fearful or worrisome thoughts. This is helpful in real danger, but sometimes our bodies get confused and react this way to harmless situations. These patterns may not make sense to the mind, but they do to the body, and we may need a little help to return to a calm and safe state.

You have the power to reassure your body and restore a sense of safety within. You can help your system return to balance and homeostasis (the ventral vagal state of the autonomic nervous system), where you feel ease, steadiness, and centered. When feeling this ease, your ability to be social and connect with others (social engagement system) feels more natural, leaving you to feel a sense of safety and connection in your environment and with others.

If arousal is unaddressed, your body will attempt to preserve its energy through downregulating into a conservation state (dorsal vagal division of the autonomic nervous system), leading to fatigue, overwhelm, and dissociation. In this state you may feel immobilized and adrift. Becoming familiar with your internal energy shifts can help your body feel acknowledged and attended to, allowing it the opportunity to return to a state of safety.

Noticing and Naming Your Shifting Internal Energy Flow

Autonomic shifts occur throughout the day and typically happen unconsciously, but we can learn to pay attention to them consciously. Deb Dana, a clinician and one of the leading teachers of polyvagal theory, calls becoming aware of these states "noticing and naming."[4] This reflection will awaken your neuroception and help you recognize energy shifts in your autonomic nervous system through directing your attention to changes in your energy levels—your flows of energy—in response to your body and environment.

- Take a moment to notice your environment. Focus your attention on something pleasant around you and consider what makes it pleasing. Observe how your body's energy shifts and responds to this enjoyable aspect of your environment. For example, as I write, my small dog is lying at my feet. I notice a smile comes to my face as my body feels the warmth of her fur on my feet and legs. I also notice an internal flow of calming energy. Try to describe as specifically as possible how your body responds to what you notice.

- Recall a social interaction that irritated you. What specifically was irritating about it? How did you know you were irritated? Notice how your body's energy shifted and responded to this unpleasant social interaction. For example, I recall an interaction with my spouse in which I felt misunderstood. My body responded with tension in my shoulders and a quickening heartbeat. Internally, I felt a surge of energy and heat. Try to describe as specifically as possible how your body responded to this irritation.

- Recall a social interaction that felt pleasing and safe to you. What made this interaction feel this way? How did you know you felt safe and at ease? Notice how your body's energy shifts in response to this pleasing and safe social interaction. For example, I remember taking a walk with a friend. I felt connected, and my body responded by feeling an overall sense of release, peace, and joy. Internally, my energy felt grounded and steady. Try to describe as specifically as possible how your body responded to this moment of safety.

Moving forward, I encourage you to start noticing how your body's energy shifts and changes according to what's happening in your environment, when you are around others, and even with food. Ask: *What do I notice inside?* Each time you notice and name what's happening, you build interoceptive awareness and help your nervous system anchor back to safety.

EMBODIED PRACTICE

Your Body as a Canvas

PART TWO: AN INTEROCEPTIVE MOMENT

The more you engage with your body's communication system and begin to understand its signals (through interoception), the better you can help your nervous system regulate and restore balance. Your body wants to be listened to and cared for, in the same way you feel seen and validated when someone truly listens to you. Attentiveness can bring a shift in energy, a change in breath, or muscle relaxation.

This practice, which builds on the previous Your Body as a Canvas practice, strengthens the connection between interoception and your nervous system. It helps you develop a new language and relationship with your body through sensory listening as you explore how energy flows differently depending on your nervous system's sense of safety. Listening requires two key components: pausing and slowing down so your body can process messages and your response to them. This will help you develop a richer, more nuanced language around your bodily sensations and lay the foundation for a new response to them.

1. Revisit part one of this practice, where you identified the body locations for specific exceptional experiences. Choose one of those body locations to work with now.

2. Sit comfortably and take a few breaths. Close your eyes or soften your gaze.

3. Place a hand on the area. Remember that touch helps your body feel seen and acknowledged.

4. Sense what the area feels like. Is it tight or tense, hard or soft? As if you could see inside your body, what do you notice inside this area? Describe it.

5. Does your body associate this sensation with safety or lack of safety?

6. Notice any shift in your internal energy as you bring attention to this area.

7. With your hand on the area, gently increase the pressure of your touch and repeat: *I sense you and I feel you.* See if you can stay with whatever comes up, noticing, naming, and repeating the words.

8. After a few minutes, check in. Has anything shifted? Does it feel less tense? Do you feel a sense of returning to your center?

Practice with each area you discovered in part one of the exercise. Notice how your body responds to being seen, named, and touched. Ignoring your body's communication can increase fearful thoughts and leave your body feeling like an enemy. Attending to sensations calms what feels unsafe and creates opportunities for repair and connection.

Learning to Recognize Dysregulation

Exceptional experiences can shape how our nervous and sensory systems perceive danger, even long after the event. Our bodies learn from these experiences and later react to similar situations as if they were equally dangerous.

When your body detects danger it activates the stress response (sympathetic), releasing hormones, such as adrenaline and cortisol, that keep you on high alert and create dysregulation in your nervous system. Without recognizing and addressing these changes, you may drift further from your center, feeling stuck in unsafety and unease. This can confuse you and lead to blaming yourself and your body.

Dysregulation disrupts interoceptive signals, making them hard to identify or understand. Support your body by noticing and naming dysregulation and reconnecting with your sensory cues.

EMBODIED REFLECTION

What It's Like Inside When You Are in Your Center

Let's get familiar with what it's like when you're centered—steady, grounded, and connected. This often indicates that your nervous system is in the ventral vagal state. If you're unfamiliar with this as an ongoing experience, consider even a fleeting moment of ground-edness—recall perhaps a moment of comfort or joy.

- Recall a moment when you felt grounded and comfortable.

- When you're in your center, what happens in your body? How does your body let you know?

- How would you describe it: ease, release, openness, peace, safety, balanced energy, aliveness?

- Are your muscles loose? Is your heartbeat soft? Is your breath free? List the sensations that you can observe.

- What happens to your mind when you are centered? Is it clear, calm, and focused? Do you feel curious and alert? Steady and open? Are there any other words you would use to describe this state of mind?

- Are you familiar with this internal experience? How often does your body return to this state?

Sensing this steady state may be challenging, but even small moments—what Deb Dana refers to as "glimmers"—are available to you.[5] Your body remembers homeostasis, calm, safety, and connection. Even if you experienced these feelings only briefly, imagine this was once your natural state. Your body can remember what once felt good, not just what didn't. It remembers comfort, joy, and belonging—even if it's been a while.

When we are not centered, dysregulation can feel like our energy shifts into overdrive or underdrive. The following reflections will help you become familiar with both states.

What It's Like Inside When You Are in Overdrive

When your body senses danger it activates the sympathetic response, triggering the fight, flight, or freeze response. This can feel like your energy shifting into overdrive, causing increased heart rate, rapid breathing, heightened blood pressure, and the release of stress hormones like adrenaline and cortisol. Each person's experience varies; for me, it starts with a racing heart and shortness of breath that leads to a cloudy mind and feelings of agitation.

Let's get familiar with what it's like when you're off-center—activated, in overdrive, ungrounded. This internal feeling may mean your internal body has shifted into the sympathetic nervous system, or a state of hyperarousal.

- Remember the last time you felt anxious or agitated.

- When in overdrive, what happens in your body?

- How would you describe it? Is there tension or holding? Does your body feel shaky, energized, alive, frightened, or agitated or alarmed?

- What are some of your body's signals that you're in this state? Do you have sweaty palms, shaky hands, or a racing heart? Is your breath constricted or shallow? List the internal sensations that stand out the most to you.

- What happens to your mind in this state? Is it clear and focused, confused or cloudy, slow and dull, or fast and speedy? Are there any other words you would use to describe this state of mind?

- Is this internal experience familiar? How old is it?
  When did it start?

- If it is unfamiliar, have you ever felt like this?
  When does it occur?

The next time you notice your energy shifting into overdrive, pause and take a deep breath. Gently move your body by swaying or rocking, and name that you are off your middle. Return to the Finding Your Center practice (page 100) to remember what centering feels like.

What It's Like Inside When You Are in Underdrive

Unlike sympathetic activation, which ramps up your system into overdrive, dorsal activation slows everything down into underdrive. Your heart rate, breathing, and blood pressure decrease as your body conserves energy. In this protective state I often feel heavy, sad, and alone, my mind filled with worry and ruminating thoughts.

Let's explore what it's like when you're off-center—depleted, in underdrive, ungrounded. This may mean your system has shifted into a dorsal vagal state of hypoarousal.

- When in underdrive, what happens in your body? How does your body signal this state?

- How would you describe it? As dullness, listlessness, shutdown, collapse, or pain?

- What are the first signals? Do you feel stuck, immobilized, have a racing heart, or shallow breath?

- What happens to your mind—is it cloudy, confused, slow, or fast?

- Is this internal experience familiar? How old is it? When did it start?

- If unfamiliar, have you ever felt like this? When does it occur?

When you notice your energy shifting into underdrive, take a deep breath, move, sway, or rock, and name it as being off your middle. Return to the Finding Your Center practice (page 100) to sense your middle.

Finding Your Natural Balance

When centered, your body returns to safety and ease, and you feel yourself again. This is where you experience joy, peace, compassion, and connection on an embodied level. It's common to feel you rarely reach this state or to question if you ever have—that's okay, as you are here to help your body learn how to experience this center more often.

Your neurobiological development and nervous system are unique. You came into the world leaning toward one state more than the other, and your nervous system may have had other attributes from the beginning, such as sensory-processing or sensory-integration issues, attention deficit disorder, autism spectrum disorders, or brain trauma at birth. This natural range of differences in how our nervous systems work is what is referred to as neurodiversity. As you grew up and accumulated exceptional experiences, your natural inclinations interacted with your life experiences and shaped your nervous system's ability to shift its internal states. Although this may be the case, we each also possess the ability to relearn sensory skills and help our nervous system rebalance back to safety.

EMBODIED REFLECTION

What Kind of Nervous System Did I Arrive With?

> I needed a deeper understanding, a knowing
> on the level of the inside of my body.
> **—Jean-Marie, study participant**

Reflecting on your unique system is crucial for developing a new understanding of how your energy shifts and flows.

- Did you come into the world leaning toward overdrive, easily moved off-center into a state of fear, anger, panic, or worry?

- Did you come into the world leaning toward underdrive, easily moved off-center into a state of depression, helplessness, shame, or numbness?

- Did you come into the world centered, until that state shifted based on your life experiences?

Even if you naturally lean toward one state more than the other, you can help your body experience, even briefly, a return to center, where your heart beats rhythmically with variation and ease and your breath is fluid, free, and open. Your body remembers feeling relaxed and no longer in survival mode. It has a memory of safety and connection. Changing your internal experience takes time, but not as much time as you think. The more you consistently remind your body of these states of calm, the more it remembers how it wants to live.

Shifting Your State and Your Perception

Joy often emerges when we are in a balanced state. In chapter 2 you practiced embodied joy over body image (page 62). When you are balanced it's easier to shift away from seeing your body solely as an image. Stress, habits, or body oppression and marginalization can pull you away from this balanced state and into dysregulation.

Paying attention to your shifting internal states throughout the day can help you become curious about how your perception of your body changes. Reflect on the following questions to notice how your perception changes in relation to your internal state.

- How do you relate to your body when you are in overdrive? Can you feel and sense your body, or can you only see it as an image in this state?

- How do you relate to your body when you are in underdrive? Can you feel and sense your body, or can you only see it as an image in this state?

- How do you relate to your body when you are centered? Can you feel and sense your body, or can you only see it as an image in this state?

When you are dysregulated it's harder to feel connected to your body—perception becomes skewed and unreliable. In these moments, gently sway or rock, acknowledge the disembodied moment, identify your internal state, and know that, until you return to a balanced state, any image will be skewed and it is not fair to judge your body.

Women are especially familiar with the challenges of reembodying. Hormonal changes throughout life impact autonomic stability.

Dr. Lara Briden, a naturopathic doctor specializing in women's health, notes that fluctuating progesterone affects our brains and nervous systems, reducing our ability to cope with stress.[6] It's not just mood—our whole internal state shifts. This is a lot to manage, month after month, year after year.

Coping with these changes requires awareness and a consistent effort to regain our center when we lose it. Without compassionate understanding and the capacity for self-regulation, shifts in body weight or shape due to hormonal changes can disturb our body image. In these moments, we're vulnerable to diet culture and marketing, which urge us to fix our surface bodies when what we really need is safety, connection, belonging, and inner peace.

Take a moment to acknowledge the unique challenges the female body faces in attempting to reembody and to honor that embodiment is a radical act.

The Way Your Body Has Received Food

There was likely a time when you received nourishment in a calm and attentive way. Consider what happens when you try to feed a baby while moving quickly. When my daughter was born, I noticed that if I tried to feed her while chasing after my twin boys, she would become fussy and cry until I slowed down and focused on her. Babies may not consciously understand that being fed calmly feels better, but they instinctively respond to it, guided only by their internal sensations and what feels most natural to their bodies.

Your body hasn't forgotten this. Receiving food calmly is still what feels most natural and best to your body. When centered, your organs function well, digestion is optimal, and hunger and fullness signals are clear. Achieving this state at every meal isn't always possible, but the more you reflect on and become curious about your internal state around food, the easier it becomes.

Your Internal State and Food

The next time you are about to eat, ask yourself the following questions:

- *What do I notice happening inside?*

- *Am I in overdrive, underdrive, or centered?*

- *What happens if I pause and slow down?*

- *How often am I centered when I am eating? When was the last time? Was I alone or with others? What was my body doing?*

- Even if you're not centered, remember: *Even if I can't feel this now, my body still remembers the way it used to be.*

The Interdependence of Sensation, Emotion, and Thought

Disembodiment teaches us to believe we can isolate emotions and thoughts in the mind, ignoring the body's experience and the interconnectedness of emotions and body. The Buddhist concept of interdependence says all experiences are linked—nothing exists in isolation. When you feel, your body feels. Each emotion triggers a sensory response, leading to thoughts and feelings in constant interaction with your environment. This is called "embodied cognition."

Embodied cognition, drawing from philosophy, neuroscience, and psychology, offers an alternative to the traditional cognitive view by recognizing that our bodies are not just passive receivers of our mind's thoughts but active, integral parts of our cognition and emotions. Your emotions influence how your body feels and the thoughts you have, just as physical pain can affect your emotions and thoughts. Although it's not a spiritual construct, embodied cognition is analogous to the *interdependence* of your body and mind. You are one interdependent, continuous loop whereby sensations, emotions, and thoughts co-occur, even if you are unaware of this process. Sensations, emotional experiences, and thoughts are all part of this interconnectedness. There is no separation.

Sensations and emotions share a unique relationship. When one is present the other often accompanies it, whether we recognize that connection in the moment. It's common for emotions to surface after the body releases tension. You may have experienced this if you've ever had a massage or taken a yoga class and had tears well up while resting in Savasana. This sensory release shows that as your body tension eases, your nervous system returns to a more balanced state. In this centered place, emotions can be felt without becoming overwhelming.

Moving closer to our emotions can be challenging, especially if you're accustomed to the protective habit of distancing yourself from them. A typical response I hear from clients is, "If I feel my feelings, I won't be able to do anything else," or "If I let myself cry, I'll never stop!" But the truth is, emotions—like sensations—come and go. This is simply the nature of our bodies. There's a Buddhist term I appreciate, *vedana*, which refers to the arising and passing of all sensations and emotions. They will all emerge and eventually fade away. Unfortunately, our minds often mislead us, particularly during times of emotional dysregulation, making us believe that a particular sensation or feeling will last forever. Unlike our minds, however, our bodies do not understand forever. They exist in the moment and are constantly shifting and changing.

The nature of emotions in our bodies is no different. Our bodies don't want to block, build up, or hold on to emotions. Instead, they yearn for whatever you are feeling—even pleasant sensations—to flow naturally, like your breath or heartbeat. The following reflection will help you embrace this new understanding of emotions.

A River of Emotions

This practice is available as an audio recording at www.shambhala.com/body-forgiveness-practices. It has two parts and uses imagery to help you explore the nature of emotions within your body. You can practice both parts together or separately at different times. Choose any position that feels comfortable: standing, sitting, or lying down.

PART ONE

1. Close your eyes or soften your gaze.

2. Call to mind the image of a flowing river. If that's difficult to picture, feel free to find a video of one—having a clear visual is important for this practice.

3. Notice how the river flows, how it moves over, under, around, and between anything in its way. It may slow down, but it does not stop.

Your emotions want to move in the same way. Like water in a river, emotions flow, slow down, and find their way again—rising, falling, weaving in and out, above and below, and in between anything in its way. Even strong emotions follow the same natural rhythm.

PART TWO

1. Take a breath and choose an emotion that tends to be challenging for you—one that you might label as "unpleasant."

2. Imagine this emotion moving along your internal river.

3. How does this emotion move inside your body? Does it get stuck somewhere? Notice if there is a place where it seems to stick, dam up, or slow down before moving again.

4. Can it find its way over, under, around, or through anything in its path?

5. If it feels stuck or blocked, take another breath and gently move that part of your body to see if the emotion can begin to flow again.

Take a moment to reflect on how you've dealt with unpleasant emotions in the past. Imagine letting these emotions become part of the ever-changing river of your experiences. You may notice that your body tends to react to intense emotions, such as sadness, loneliness, grief, anger, disappointment, frustration, or shame, by either becoming excessively energized (overdrive) or shutting down (underdrive). When this happens, your emotional flow is likely damming up.

Think about what happens when a river is dammed: The water becomes stagnant, toxic substances can build up, and the river loses its vitality, disrupting the entire ecosystem. The same is true for your emotions and body. When emotions aren't allowed to flow, we become increasingly dysregulated and disconnected from ourselves. Embracing a new, more fluid way of being with challenging emotions is essential—it feels natural to your body's rhythm and honors its interdependent nature.

As we conclude this chapter, I hope you have gained a deeper understanding and appreciation for the incredible effort your internal system has put into making sense of exceptional experiences and keeping you safe. Even though it may not feel like it in the moment, your body moving into overdrive and underdrive has only been to protect you. It's important to acknowledge that there is a reason your relationship with your body has been so complicated for so long. As you begin to notice, name, and acknowledge your internal experience, your body will begin to gift you by responding in a new, more centered way.

> I now understand my body was just trying to protect me.
> —MAGGIE, STUDY PARTICIPANT

> My body had no intent to harm me. It's a two-way process.
> I had to have the willingness to understand what's there.
> —MEG, STUDY PARTICIPANT

Embodying

go now *dear friend*
and journey on
ask your heart what it wants
and give it just that
—ZÖE LAWRIE

WELCOME TO PART TWO. In part one we explored our disembodied world, the impact upon our internal states, and the difficulties they create for our bodies, especially for women seeking to reconnect with themselves. You learned about embodiment and the steps needed to return to a sense of wholeness, including understanding your body's unique sensory language. You and your body are learning this language together, step by step, and it can be challenging. You opened to curiosity and developed a deeper understanding about the many reasons you lost connection with your body.

Now, in part two, we enter a relational experience between you and your body where you begin to truly listen to what your body has been trying to communicate. Your body has been waiting for you to give it a chance. Giving your body a chance means cultivating self-compassion—your greatest ally on the journey to reembodiment. It involves allowing your body to feel everything it feels, including emotions like grief, regret, and shame. Ultimately it is about understanding and embracing what it means to forgive your body.

5

EMBODYING COMPASSION

Giving Your Body a Chance

The human body is already and always abiding in the
meditative state, the domain of awakening—and we
are just trying to gain entry.[1]
—REGINALD RAY

I wasn't born with criticisms.
—JADE, STUDY PARTICIPANT

I'm a human BEING.
—JOAN, STUDY PARTICIPANT

THE FIFTH STAGE of body forgiveness is learning to embody compassion. In this chapter you'll discover how self-compassion deep-
ens your connection to your body by inviting you to approach, listen
to, and understand it in a new way. Rather than seeing your body as
just an object, this chapter encourages you to engage with it fully.
Now is the time to become curious about what your body can teach
you. When you give your body a chance to be heard, you'll find it has
valuable insights to share.

The Relationship Between Self-Compassion and Forgiveness

Years ago, during my first qualitative research study on self-compassion and eating-disorder recovery, I found a significant connection between forgiveness and self-compassion. Some participants reported forgiveness came first and made self-compassion possible, while others experienced self-compassion first, which then opened the door to forgiveness. Later I realized that those who felt that forgiveness came first were often relating to forgiveness on a mental level, feeling they had done something wrong. (You'll read more about this in chapter 7.)

Fast forward ten years to my current research on forgiveness and embodiment. I asked, "What is your experience with self-compassion and forgiveness toward your body?" This time, everyone agreed: Self-compassion had to come first before forgiveness could flourish. Forgiveness was described as coming from the heart, nourished by self-compassion. Through this journey, I learned that to achieve embodiment—a subjective, lived relationship with your body—self-compassion is essential. It's what allows you to meet, hold, support, and soothe yourself, and to maintain a relationship with your body over time.

Compassion Is Inherent in Your Body

The late Vietnamese Buddhist teacher Thich Nhat Hanh offered the perfect teaching story to show how compassion is inherent to the body. Imagine how you would react if you were walking barefoot down the street and stepped on a nail. Immediately, and without conscious thought, your hand would reach down to embrace and comfort the injured foot. Your body does not require any discussion or deliberation ahead of this response. One part of your body instinctively responds to another part that is in pain. You don't need to take time to think about whether you deserve care; your body simply acts. This is the natural compassion inherent within us. Each organ supports the others, always striving for optimum functionality and balance. Your body wants to protect and nurture, just as it wants to be protected and cared for.

Developing care and compassion for our bodies isn't always easy. If this has been difficult for you, you may already understand some of the reasons why. When we disconnect from our bodies, we forget their natural compassion. Like any long-term relationship, we can neglect to appreciate what our bodies do for us every day. Instead of nurturing a compassionate partnership, we may fall into adversarial or even contemptuous relational dynamics. Just as criticism and disdain can damage any relationship, it can also harm your relationship with your body. Before we can foster a new, compassionate understanding of this relationship, let's first explore self-compassion and why it's so essential for healing.

When I teach about compassion for others, I use this embodied definition: *Compassion* is when your heart trembles in response to someone else's pain and suffering. Take a moment to consider this. Compassion doesn't come from the mind; it arises in the body, often as a movement or energy in your heart center. This is why we feel our hearts ache when we see someone suffering.

Self-compassion is the same trembling of the heart, but in response to your own pain and suffering. This can be challenging, as many of us are practiced at empathizing with others but struggle to extend that same kindness to ourselves. So, for now, I'm not asking you to feel your heart tremble for your own pain—just stay open and curious about what self-compassion might look, sound, or feel like.

Three Key Components of Self-Compassion

Kristin Neff, a leading self-compassion researcher, describes three interconnected components of self-compassion: common humanity, mindfulness, and self-kindness.[2] Our common humanity helps us recognize our struggles as part of the larger human experience, so we feel less isolated in our suffering. Mindfulness is about maintaining balanced awareness of painful thoughts and feelings rather than getting swept away by them. Self-kindness means replacing harsh self-criticism with understanding and compassion. Self-compassion might feel distant or unattainable at times, but many of us practice it more often than we realize—we just may not be aware of it. Let's look at these three components and how they relate to your relationship with your body.

Finding Common Humanity with Other Women

Common humanity begins with the shared experience of having a female body in this world. My research participants expressed this in many ways:

- MAGGIE: "I kept believing I'd done something wrong and that I was wrong."

- SARAH: "I was so hypersensitive out there. My body just always wanted to escape."

- AMELIA: "It was exhausting and left me scared of my body."

- SOPHIA: "The external view was the pain my body had to endure."

- PEARL: "It wasn't my idea to hate my body."

- JADE: "Everywhere I look, someone is suffering from this! Everyone is struggling—my friends, my family members. Why is it that when I see a picture of myself, the joy is ripped away from me? How did that happen?"

You may relate to these statements, which reflect the shared suffering of women's bodies in a disembodied world. This is not yours alone—it's been felt by many generations.

When I lead women's embodiment retreats, we share not only our own stories of pain and suffering but also those of our mothers and grandmothers. Our bodies absorb messages from the world, as well as the feelings and experiences of the women before us. I call this "intergenerational absorption." The time to protect your body and stop this cycle of hatred and harm is now. Many women want to stop this cycle for their daughters and granddaughters, and understanding intergenerational absorption can help.

You already know how you've absorbed messages from the world. But to develop more self-compassion, it's important to reflect on the messages you received from the women around you—who themselves absorbed messages from those around them, creating a cycle that's lasted for generations. For example, the first known diet book, *The Art of Living Long*, by Luigi Cornaro, was published in 1558, around the same time the mind-body divide took hold in Western thought. Thinness became prioritized in the 1800s, promoting a view of beauty that emphasized appearance, reinforced the mind-body duality, and reduced the body to merely an image. Before this, diet culture mainly centered around the idea that the ideal body belonged to white, Western men. But as women's rights advocates began to challenge the patriarchal belief that slim, strong bodies—and the self-control they symbolized—were exclusively for men, they encouraged white women to pursue the same ideal. This push for thinness became both a form of resistance against patriarchal control and a way to distinguish themselves from working-class immigrants and Black women, who were unfairly stereotyped as overweight and lacking discipline. As a result, diet culture's messages have primarily targeted privileged white women for centuries while oppressing and marginalizing women of color and those with less privilege.[3]

Your Body's Family Tree

This reflection encourages you to consider how the women who came before you were impacted by these messages. It is designed to deepen your understanding of our common humanity and to cultivate kindness. It is inspired by assignments I had in both undergraduate and graduate training to create a family tree to explore my lineage. Here, we will focus specifically on how your ancestors' relationships with their bodies relates to your relationship with your body today. Each woman's journey has been uniquely challenging. Trace back as many generations as you can. Some stories will be familiar; others will have been passed down through family lore.

As you write, consider what body messages you absorbed from each woman. When you finish, share your reflections with at least two other women. Sharing these stories fosters connection and self-compassion. Notice when your body or mind feels at capacity—then pause and return later if needed.

Choose a woman from your lineage (maternal or paternal) and use the following prompts to guide you. If it was someone you knew, write from your own observations. If it was an ancestor you never met, write from family history or what you may be able to surmise based on what you know about the time and circumstances of their life.

- What did you sense or feel (or what do you imagine you would have sensed or felt) when around their body?

- What did you witness, or what do you imagine their relationship with their body was like?

- What did you observe about their body, or what could you assume, that was beyond body image?

- What messages do you believe you absorbed from them?

Here is an example of my reflection on my own life, tracing back the body messages I absorbed from three generations of maternal ancestors.

MY MATERNAL GREAT-GRANDMOTHER

She was known as Big Nana, and I only knew her through pictures. She was still alive when I was born, and the story goes that she sat in her rocking chair and rocked every great-grandchild until she passed away. The photos of her show long, feminine hair that she wore in a bun. She had a stern expression, but a slight smile on her face. Her body was large and robust, exuding a sense of safety and protection. I can only imagine her relationship with her body as one of embodied grace and strength rather than one focused on image. But who knows? Was she somehow shielded from societal messages? I like to think so. Even her name suggested a sense of protection. I imagine that I absorbed her strength, grace, and "largeness" from the brief time I spent in her arms. Is this the protection I returned to once I reembodied? I wonder.

MY MATERNAL GRANDMOTHER

Despite her reluctance for the job, I knew her to be my second mother. She seemed unhappy most of the time, and I could feel her unhappiness within myself whenever I was around her, which was often. Her body appeared old, frail, and weak long before its time. In later years I came to understand that she had been medically ill for most of her life. Her kidneys failed suddenly at a young age due to a medical error. Her body constantly struggled to maintain stability through her heart, lungs, and kidney functions. She endured breast cancer and underwent a full mastectomy that left her with lifelong lymphedema. As a child I didn't pay attention to her body size; I was only aware of its suffering. I don't believe she focused much on her size either. Instead, she was consumed with the fight for survival in a body that I can only imagine felt like a betrayal. I recall her pushing herself to cook and clean daily for seven people, likely ignoring what her body was trying to communicate to her. I imagine I absorbed a sense of fear, perhaps even terror, that one's body could turn against you at any moment. This helped me understand why, as a teenager, I felt the need to hold on to a body that wouldn't change. I also learned the importance of pushing through the body's sensory experience to survive. This mindset was especially valued in my family, particularly among the women.

MY MOTHER

As I wrote this chapter, my mother was ninety-three, suffering from end-stage dementia. She passed before I finished this book. My mother was the caregiver for everyone around her. She took care of her ailing mother, her alcoholic husband, and her three children, all while running a business she never wanted. Throughout my life I watched her body change shape, which seemed to correlate with the quality of her life and her relationship with food. She often grabbed food on the go and would scrape our plates to consume the leftovers. I remember feeling anxious around her, especially during meals, as I could sense her energy shifting into overdrive while eating. It was hard for her to breathe and eat at the same time, and I wanted her to be able to breathe easily. As her life experiences became heavier and more painful—losing her parents and dealing with a sick husband—her body grew larger. She expressed her unhappiness about this, and my father would tease her about her size. I felt her emotional and physical pain and wished he would stop.

This was the 1980s when diet culture surged to reach an all-time high. She, along with those around her, viewed her body with feelings of disgust and criticism, believing it was not okay that her body exceeded the ideal body image of that time. I absorbed the message that any change to my body, especially if it meant gaining weight, was unacceptable. Fat was equated with distress and unacceptability. I learned that my image was equivalent to acceptance and whether I would be okay and loved. I absorbed the message to stay thin at all costs, as the alternative was too painful. I also absorbed the lesson that I had to push through my body's signals to survive, and that it was necessary to care for others above yourself and your body. I am sure she absorbed this from her mother, and her mother from Big Nana. It was no surprise to me that at age sixteen, when my world changed through exceptional experiences and diet culture ruled outside and inside my home, restricting my food intake seemed like a reasonable and helpful alternative to alleviate the pain my body was experiencing.

As you complete your reflection, check in. What do you notice inside? This is a good time to revisit the Your Body as a Canvas practice from chapter 4 and notice where these absorbed messages may live in your body. Can you bring a hand, pillow, or blanket to soften and soothe that area? Maybe add some gentle movement. Your body has held on to these messages for generations—it's tired of carrying them.

As I reflect on the intergenerational messages my body carries, I feel sensations concentrated along my right side, from my neck down to my leg. I hold both sides of my neck and sway to soothe myself. Once I return to center, I sense my heart tremble and my compassion deepen for my grandmother, my mother, and myself—acknowledging the years of pain and suffering that our bodies have endured. Can you feel your heart tremble in response to these intergenerational messages? Maybe tears come. I'm sorry that you and the women in your life have carried this burden for so long and that your body has held on to this pain.

Cultivating Mindfulness of Your Body

Mindfulness is being present to whatever you're experiencing. Jon Kabat-Zinn defines it as being aware, nonjudgmentally and on purpose, in the present moment.[4] Like compassion, mindfulness is inherent to our bodies. Our bodies are designed to exist in the present, experiencing life as it unfolds—like young children, who approach everything with wonder and a fresh perspective. But our minds often dwell on the past or worry about the future, distorting our experiences along with the sensations in our bodies. Instead of staying grounded in the present, our thoughts can take over, leading to rumination about past experiences or future anxieties. This disconnect can create confusion, self-criticism, and feelings of being unsafe. Self-criticism not only damages self-worth but also triggers your nervous system's threat response. Your body interprets self-criticism as danger, which leads to a cycle of shame, hopelessness, and disconnection—a cycle many of us know well.

Mindfulness helps break this cycle by creating space around self-critical thoughts, allowing your body to be seen and felt, and allowing other parts of you to emerge. Consider the part of you that picked up this book, eager to connect with your body in a new way. Approach this part with curiosity and kindness. If you've done any practices from part one, you've already practiced mindfulness by being present with your sensations, slowing down, and creating space for curiosity to bloom.

Trying to learn new things in a mind filled with blame or shame leads to nervous-system dysregulation and makes it hard for your brain to process new information, especially sensory information. Think of a teacher who attempted to motivate through criticism—how much did you really learn in that environment? In contrast, learning with curiosity and kindness is energizing and encouraging. There is a reason you enjoyed attending classes with teachers who created a safe and supportive environment. The same is true for your body and brain during moments of kindness. Recognizing a self-critical thought (through mindfulness) creates space to witness it and acknowledge and accept what you just noticed without judging or criticizing. It gives you the space to become curious about the thought rather than attaching to or believing it. This balanced approach helps you cultivate and maintain new learning.

One study participant, Sophia, spoke about the energy she needed to stay present: "Initially, I was trying hard to be present. It felt like I was forcing myself to be present all the time, which isn't necessary. Instead, it's about the energy behind the effort." I appreciate Sophia's insight—it's not about being forceful but about finding a balance between engagement and ease. Imagine approaching your body with genuine intent to listen. Just showing up with the intention to listen—regardless of how successful you feel—represents a significant shift.

EMBODIED PRACTICE

The Energy of Being Present

This practice is available as an audio recording at www.shambhala.com/body-forgiveness-practices. It will show you how to be present with yourself without trying too hard.

1. Find a comfortable seated position, ideally with support behind you. Imagine an invisible string extending upward from below your navel to help you sense your center.

2. Gently sway or rock your body, embracing the pillars of slowing down and stillness that are needed for mindful awareness. If you wish, you can continue the gentle rocking or swaying as you transition into the following steps.

3. Place your hands on either side of your head. Feel the gentle pressure of your hands and repeat: *May I show up with the*

full intent to be present to the sensation of touch to my head and what I notice right in this moment. Allow the quality of your energy to be moderate.

4. Place your hands on either side of your neck. Feel the gentle pressure of your hands and repeat: *May I show up with the full intent to be present to the sensation of touch to my neck and what I notice right in this moment.* Allow the quality of your energy to be moderate.

5. Place your hands on either side of your torso and repeat: *May I show up with the full intent to be present to the sensation of touch to my side body and what I notice right in this moment.* Allow the quality of your energy to be moderate.

6. Pause to notice if your mind has run away into thoughts about your body as an image or if it is busy criticizing instead of focusing on sensations. If so, pause the practice and gently move your body, label the thought as unkind and unwholesome to your body and mind, and come back into the practice when you're centered again.

7. Place a hand on top of each leg, gently press, and repeat: *May I show up with the full intent to be present to the sensation of touch to my leg and what I notice right in this moment.*

Use this practice throughout the day, even if you focus on just one area. As your attention grows, you may find it helpful when self-critical moments arise, creating space to gently return to your body.

Discovering Self-Kindness for Your Body

By reading this book and seeking to understand your body in a new way, you're already being kind to yourself. Recognizing the small steps you are taking is a foundation for self-kindness. You began exploring kindness through our common humanity in part one, focusing on disembodiment and what it means to be disembodied in the world. Recognizing that disembodiment affects all bodies, though some more than others, fosters self-kindness. It acknowledges that this is hard and that disembodiment was never your intention. Understanding your body's unique experiences and your internal reactions is an act of self-kindness.

Fifteen years ago I had an oophorectomy (removal of one ovary). I worried about how my body would adapt, but my doctor, who was kind and very in tune with the body, reassured me that my body would instinctively know what to do. I found this idea both relieving and astonishing—different parts of our bodies work together to support one another. Organs, joints, and muscles collaborate in one interconnected, compassionate system. That's the thing: Compassion and kindness are your body's nature.

Unfortunately, many of us overlook this until something goes wrong. Disembodiment rarely helps us to develop kindness toward our bodies. Instead it makes us forget the true nature of our bodies, leaving us disconnected and unaware of all they do for us. You're not alone in forgetting about your body. Many people—including me—have pushed their bodies to extremes or neglected them, thinking we needed to change our body's health, ability, or size to fit in. You're not the only one who has criticized or shamed your body or believed it was the source of your problems. Remembering you're not alone fosters self-kindness, which helps self-compassion grow. Self-compassion responds with understanding: *I did the best I could,* and *How could I have known otherwise?*

How Could I Not?

The goal of self-compassion is to cultivate a new, softer, kinder perspective on familiar thoughts rather than to eliminate them. The more we can meet these repetitive thoughts in a new way, the more they will fade into the background over time. This practice helps you develop a gentler understanding of your journey with your body. As you read the passage below, place a hand on your heart or another soothing area. Gently close your eyes or keep a soft gaze, and repeat each phrase as if you're sitting next to your body, saying these words to it:

1. How could I not have absorbed the messages telling me to change you, shift you, and make you something different than how you wished to be?

2. How could I not have absorbed the messages telling me to treat you unkindly and to believe my ideas and thoughts knew more than you did?

3. How could I not have absorbed the messages telling me to criticize, blame, and shame you?

4. How could I not have absorbed the messages telling me to push you to do things that don't feel natural or good to you?

5. How could I not have absorbed the messages telling me to ignore what you have been trying to tell me all along?

6. How could I not?

Take a deep breath and notice how the words resonate within you. What shifts when you embrace a self-compassionate understanding of what you and your body have experienced? Notice any changes in your body, mind, or energy. Your nervous system appreciates your willingness to acknowledge and process this truth.

When I was a teenager my life changed dramatically after my father's traumatic death, which led to the development of an eating disorder. I believed the eating disorder was my fault, a notion reinforced by my mother's gynecologist when I stopped menstruating. He scolded me, saying I was purposefully harming my mother by not eating. His harsh words filled me with anger, made me feel voiceless, and only deepened my self-criticism and hatred—until I eventually found the strength to reject those hurtful messages.

As my self-compassion grew, I realized I never asked for this. That's the truth for me and for you. You never asked to feel unsafe in your body, or for the messages and exceptional experiences that confused your internal world. You never asked for unkindness toward yourself or your body. Self-compassion knows you never asked for it, and by repeating "I never asked for this," you reinforce the protective nature of self-compassion that stands up to self-criticism and says, "Hold on—I never wanted this for myself or my body!"

Self-Compassion as Your Body's Safe Harbor

A moment of self-compassion not only softens self-critical thoughts but also reprograms your internal system by securing the safety and protection you and your body have always longed for. In her book *Anchored*, Deb Dana calls the vagus nerve the "compassion nerve."[5] Each time you return to your center, you have the opportunity to cultivate compassion and reduce self-criticism. The more you develop self-compassion, the more it can support you during times of dysregulation, guiding you back to your center. Over time, self-compassion creates a continuous loop: Building it during calm moments helps you manage the not-so-calm ones.

Self-touch is one of the most effective ways to develop a sense of compassion, security, and protection within, as it helps to anchor your nervous system back to safety and your center. If self-touch feels awkward, it may be due to self-critical thoughts that keep you seeing your body as an image rather than a sensory experience. Or your dislike of touch may be related to the powerful emotion of shame (which we'll discuss in the next chapter). If you feel uncomfortable, gently remind yourself that touch is inherently familiar to our bodies. Remember, you never asked for shame to interfere with your ability to soothe yourself. In this next practice, I invite you to let your body experience the soothing power of self-touch, quieting your mind and allowing your body to receive.

EMBODIED PRACTICE

Soothing and Containing with Touch

Use this practice several times a day to introduce your body to comfort through soothing touch. It's natural to your body and key to building self-compassion.

1. Feel free to lie down or sit for this practice.

2. Take a release breath: Inhale through your nose, exhale through your mouth. Repeat several times.

3. Bring both hands together—palm to palm, fingers interlaced, or simply holding one hand in the other. Gently press and notice the soft pulsation.

4. Place one hand on your heart's center, the other on top of it, and gently press. Notice the pressure of your hands meeting this space.

5. Stay here with the sensation. Do you want to steady your hands, gently press, pulse, or move in a circle? Find what brings comfort and ease.

6. Close your eyes or keep a soft gaze. Let your breath join the movement of your hands, imagining your hands moving your breath. After a few minutes it may feel like your breath is moving your hands. Go with it.

7. If you feel like moving to other areas—shoulders, chest, head, neck—let yourself follow that impulse.

8. Stay until you feel a return to your center, where your mind can rest and your body feels grateful for this moment of comfort. Repeat: *This is comfort, this is ease, this is kindness.*

Notice what's happening inside after this practice. Did it help you return to your center? Did your energy shift? Notice what this shift feels like inside. Maybe you notice a softening or the river of emotions unblocking as your body responds to the overture of compassion.

EMBODIED REFLECTION

How Do I Start and End My Day: The Essential Bookends

A key way to build self-compassion is to reflect on how you begin and end each day—these are your "bookends" of embodied self-compassion.

- When you wake up, notice your first thought about your body. Is it a complaint, an annoyance, or something about your body as an image?

- What would it be like to be present in your body in a neutral way? Your body just *is*. It is here and you are here. Nothing else matters in this moment. Just be. You are both here, giving each other a chance to start the day in a new way.

- At night, as you lie down, notice your thoughts toward your body. Is there a complaint, an annoyance, or something about your body as an image? Is something from the day lingering in your mind?

- What would it be like to be present in your body in a neutral way? Your body just *is.* It is here and you are here. Nothing else matters in this moment. Just be. You are both here, giving each other a chance to end the day differently. As you rest, maybe bring in the realizations *I never asked for this* and *My body never asked for this.*

This reflection can help you bring together mindfulness and self-compassion to start and end each day, fostering a gentle, present focus and attention to your body.

Developing A Self-Compassionate Relationship with Food

In a world obsessed with food rules, we rarely see eating as an act of self-kindness. Instead, food becomes the enemy—something to fear and control. Have you ever stopped to consider how confusing food rules are for your body? Our bodies have become passive receivers of patterns that may be the opposite of kind, and this creates confusion along the way. Yes, bodies get confused!

No one is born wishing to diet or have food withheld. Your body doesn't know whether a food is good or bad until it receives it and gets to decide. Diet culture has led us far from a natural relationship with food and the kindness and nourishment our bodies intuitively crave. It's only through developing an internal conversation with your body that you can know what it truly feels. Remember, from the time you were a developing fetus to when you were born, food was kindness. Feeding yourself is self-compassionate and most natural to your body.

Developing a Kinder Relationship with Food

This reflection will help you develop a kinder relationship with food. Reflect on these questions daily and perhaps during meals—they're important for building interoceptive knowledge and, most important, self-compassion.

- Is food received in your body consistently and predictably, or is it haphazard and unpredictable? Can your body expect nourishment at least three times a day, or does it have to wait for long stretches?

- Do you ever let your body decide what foods it likes or dislikes, or are all choices made from your mind, overriding your body's communication?

- Does your body decide when it's had enough or wants more, or do those decisions come from your mind?

- At each meal remind yourself that your body once had a very different relationship with food. Can you be present in this moment, observing your body and food?

- Sense into these moments with food. What happens inside? Does your body send any sensory messages? Do these sensations feel kind and comforting? Does this moment bring you back to your center?

- If not, pause and return to the Soothing and Containing with Touch practice. After a few minutes, see what it's like to return to food in a new way, giving you, your body, and food another chance.

Self-compassion and its components—our common humanity, mindfulness, and self-kindness—are now by your side as you continue your radical path toward reembodiment. There's a reason my study participants said compassion was essential before moving into the muddy waters of intense emotions like grief, shame, and regret, which we'll explore in the next chapter. Feel free to linger with chapter 5 as long as you need to develop these essential skills. Your body thanks you for giving it a chance to experience something different: being understood through our common humanity, treated with kindness through mindful intent, and soothed through the felt sense of compassion.

6

EMBODYING GRIEF

Moving into Grieving

> Grief is a catalyst for healing. Healing grief carves the
> landscape of your heart in ways that open up deeper
> pathways of connection to others.[1]
>
> —PAULA ARAI

THE SIXTH STAGE of body forgiveness is about embodying grief. This is a new way to understand grief and allow it to move and be released within your body. Reading a whole chapter on grief takes willingness and curiosity. Grief is challenging to face but learning to navigate it is essential for forgiving your body and cultivating a more embodied relationship. To truly embody means to acknowledge grief and work toward a new relationship with it—one that is less fearful and more compassionate.

Self-compassion is essential here, and you'll want to rely on it throughout this chapter. As Kristin Neff notes, even when grief feels overwhelming, self-compassion offers a "warm embrace."[2] It can help carry you and your body through grief that's been held inside for so long. Grief left unattended often turns into fear and internal dysregulation. Self-compassion attends to grief, helping transform it from something stuck and trapped in our bodies into an active process of grieving. This process allows grief to move through us, become less frightening, and create space for forgiveness to emerge. As you'll discover, it's not just you who's been yearning to grieve— your body has been longing for this release as well.

Grief That Lives on the Inside

I call grief that manifests in the body "embodied grief." This experience is unique for each of us and is shaped by our individual nervous system and the age at which our bodies began to store grief. Still, after years of working with clients and hearing their stories, I've noticed some universal themes. Study participants and patients describe the feeling of embodied grief as heavy, weighed down, sluggish, stuck, like glue, sticky, dense, trapped, blocked, unmoving, organs weighed down, an internal cry, the need to be on the ground, curled up, and low energy.

EMBODIED REFLECTION

What Are Your Body's Words for Grief?

Pause and reflect on the words above. Do any resonate with you—not just in your mind but in your body? What does your body feel like when you experience grief? You may have your own words for embodied grief. Before you can process and move through grief, it's important to develop a less fearful relationship with this powerful emotion. The following practice will help you prepare for this journey and expand your capacity to tolerate grief's intensity.

EMBODIED PRACTICE

Circling the Edge of Grief

This practice is available as an audio recording at www.shambhala.com/body-forgiveness-practices.

1. You can do this practice sitting up or lying on your back.

2. Take a few release breaths: Lift your arms up as you inhale through your nose and let your arms swing alongside your body or stretch outward as you exhale through your mouth.

3. Which words for embodied grief stand out to you? Using the Your Body as a Canvas practice from chapter 4, imagine where you would paint these words inside your body. Where do you feel grief is trapped or stuck?

4. Place a hand, blanket, or pillow on this area. Feel the softness, warmth, and gentle pressure as you meet this area where grief lives.

   - Acknowledge it with these words: *This is grief. I see you and I feel you.*

   - Imagine this grief is encased in a circle and observe it from outside the circle. With a spirit of curiosity, what do you see and sense inside this space? How large or small is it? Does it move or stay stuck? Is there a color or texture to it? Use as many descriptive words as you can to describe the feeling of grief in your body.

   - Begin to walk the edge of the sensations of grief by using your hand to circle around the edge of the space where you feel the grief. Slowly move toward where the grief is held. Stay where it is most comfortable—neither too close nor too far. Try sending some soothing energy, like a ray of sunshine or the softness of feathers or clouds, to break up the stuck energy mass.

   - Approach this grief with balanced energy and the intention to stay present and soothe it. Take some release breaths.

   - Repeat: *This is grief. I see you, I feel you, and I can soothe you.*

You can return to this practice throughout the chapter and in daily life. Grief is often present even if we're not aware of it. It can often show up disguised as body hatred, anger, annoyance, neglect of your body's needs, fear, and especially shame and regret. Each time you notice these feelings, it's a sign that grief is present and needs attention. Taking mindful pauses and checking in with your body can help you identify embodied grief.

Blame, Betrayal, and the Body's Need for Compassion and Grieving

My research found that to shift grief into grieving, we must first navigate intense emotions like betrayal, deception, regret, and shame, along with beliefs that keep us blaming our bodies. *Body blame* means believing your body is at fault for your struggles or suffering. When you experience body blame, you may feel like a victim of your own body, as if it's let you down or caused you harm. In my study, for example, Eve said about her cancer diagnosis, "My body turned against me." Maggie recalled, "The women in the neighborhood were talking about me because of my body size. I blamed my body for years." Our bodies receive this blame, but if they could speak, they'd likely say, "I never meant to cause you harm."

You may not fully believe this yet, and that's okay. Sometimes our bodies do things that feel harmful—losing abilities, getting sick, aging, or simply not fitting in. The truth is, you didn't ask for the pain and suffering you've experienced, and neither did your body. If your body could speak, it might say, "What about me? I didn't want this either."

When we meet body blame with compassion, we can see what lies beneath—body deception. This is the shock and anguish you feel when your body turns out to be different than you expected—it is a feeling like betrayal. It can arise from any experience that changes your relationship with your body, often throwing you off-center and taking up residence as grief that remains unaddressed until another deception happens. As the study participant Eve said, her body became ill even though she felt she was doing all the right things. And Maggie shared, "I did the best I could at the time and a lot of it didn't turn out well."

I've experienced body deception many times. As a child, I was teased for being small. As a teen, I developed an eating disorder after my father died, and I wondered why my body was a source of struggle again. Hadn't it caused me enough grief as a child? I didn't realize my body wasn't causing the grief; it was trying to help me express it. The study participant Gail shared about her body's messages: "It was a somatic cry for help."

When I developed Graves' disease, what felt like body deception turned into betrayal. Even though I cared for my body, it let me down again. How could my body do this to me at a time in my life that was supposed to be the happiest? I had just given birth to my twin boys after years of struggling with infertility. Why now? Why, after I had been taking such good care of myself? I felt angry at my body again. I had long since recovered from my eating disorder and was treating my body with compassion and respect. I thought, "What does my body want from me?" The shock and pain were overwhelming. The grief weighed me down. I was exhausted, and my body begged to lie on the ground. At that moment, I didn't need answers—I just needed to be held by the earth. This position became my refuge, a practice I use myself and with clients when the grief from betrayal feels too heavy. I invite you to try this practice of grounding through grief when it feels overwhelming.

Grounding Through Grief

Recall a past body deception or betrayal—one you've known for a long time and have some understanding about. If you can do so comfortably, lie on your belly, on the ground or in bed. If that is not comfortable, sit or lie in a position where you can hold a pillow against the front of your torso, and modify the practice as needed throughout.

1. Lie on your belly. Fold your arms in front of you and rest your head on the back of your hands.

2. Roll your forehead back and forth into your arms, gently massaging this area.

3. Feel the ground supporting your front body. Soften your shoulders, chest, and belly into the ground.

4. Repeat: *The ground can hold this grief right now. The ground can hold my grief right now. I am held.*

Tears may come—if so, know that this is the river of emotions unblocking. When grief starts to move you'll feel an energy shift. It often starts deep in your belly, moving upward to your heart, throat, and eyes. Tears are your body's way of expressing emotion, signaling change and the release of hormones. When tears flow, don't fear them but acknowledge, *My body is releasing and trying to find its way back to its center.* Rest in this feeling, knowing the ground supports you and offers safety and steadiness.

I remember the tears that came as I lay on my belly, letting the ground hold me. There was pain but also the compassion I'd been cultivating for years. As I mentioned in chapter 5, self-compassion meets suffering—especially body suffering—when we allow it. For me it said, "I didn't ask for this!" And strangely, "Neither did my body!" I realized it wasn't just me suffering; my body was in pain too. We were suffering together. Compassion allowed me to see my body as part of me, sharing the suffering, not separate from it. My body wasn't purposefully doing this to me—it was longing for stability and homeostasis just as much as I was. This moment of compassion happened after grief moved into grieving and the tears flowed.

When you feel trapped and betrayed, you're in a state of overdrive or underdrive and may feel weighed down by anger, resentment, shock, or pain. If you pause and let your body be held, you can move toward center and begin to actively grieve. Study participants described the shift from feeling stuck into active grieving as shifting into a present awareness; as energy moving down, then up; and as a feeling that they were making room, opening, softening, or becoming more fluid. Many women described the movement as palms open and sweeping upward—as if grieving took the form of air, allowing their bodies to take a deep breath in and up. Some women reported spontaneously moving while sweeping their arms upward. These are the sensations of grief as it moves into grieving.

The Many Flavors of Regret

Whenever we feel our bodies have deceived or betrayed us, regret and shame, two emotions that often hide grief, are usually lurking underneath. If reading about blame and betrayal was hard, regret may be even harder. But take a breath and let compassion sit with you. First, I want to normalize regret—especially body regret. We live in a culture of toxic positivity, where slogans like "Live your life with no regrets" abound. But if you're human and have a body, you will have regrets. As embodied beings, regret is inevitable. The Buddha taught that suffering arises because we live in bodies that will get sick and die. If we're lucky, our bodies will age well, but death is inevitable. Regret is sadness or disappointment over something that happened or an opportunity that was missed. At some point, your body will disappoint you or create missed opportunities.

But regret is more than disappointment—it signals the need to mourn. When regret is strong, you can know it's grief calling for attention. Regret creates a trifecta of stuckness in our minds with the familiar refrain of would've, could've, should've. This kind of thinking pulls us into the past. Mindful awareness and self-compassion can help us return to the present. The first step is to recognize this trifecta in action. A simple acknowledgment—*There it is! Mind is stuck!*—can help bring us back to center. Self-compassion then has an opportunity to step in and remind us, "This is a moment I need to grieve. My body and I can do this together." This is how you move from feeling the sensations of stuck grief to feeling the fluidity of grieving.

Regret has multiple overlapping layers: regret from unknown and unintended experiences, regret from experiences that were known but unintended, and the muddy-water regret that often has no answers, leaving us in confusion. These layers intersect and signal your body's need to grieve. Let's look at each more closely.

UNKNOWN AND UNINTENDED REGRET

Think back to activities you loved as a child—running, playing, sports. These were fun and brought joy and aliveness to your body and spirit. But bodies change, and things we did years ago can show up later as injury or illness. For example, a friend who loved Irish dancing as a child needed emergency surgery in her fifties for a spinal injury likely caused by years of dancing. The very movements that brought her joy led to injury years later—something she couldn't have anticipated as a child. This is what we call unknown and unintended regret: "I wish I could have known." Should she regret dancing? Should she have stopped because of what might happen? These are questions born from our humanness.

Unfortunately, we can't predict our body's future. Someone else might have done the same thing and never had an issue. Bodies are different, and so there will be regrets from choices made unknowingly and unintentionally. As a yogi for over twenty-five years, I didn't know that early in my practice deep twists were destabilizing my sacroiliac joints. What I thought was helpful was actually causing harm! Years later, after pain and more anatomy training, I realized I'd been twisting incorrectly for my body. My mind rushed to would've, could've, should've. "Ugh! I wish I had known!" and "Why didn't anyone instruct me differently? I would have changed up the way I did them." This was my signal to pause, notice my stuck mind, and recognize it as a moment of grief. When self-compassion meets grief, it asks, "How could I have known?" Self-compassion softens regret, allowing grief to move into grieving.

EMBODIED REFLECTION AND PRACTICE

The Unintended and Unknown Regrets

- Reflect on the unintended and unknown regrets your body has experienced.

- List each one, and after each, repeat: *How could I have known any differently?*

- Place your hands on your lap, palms up, and sweep your arms upward toward your belly, heart, throat, and eyes. Let it be fluid.

- Sense your breath lifting inward and upward with each sweep upward, clearing space inside as grief becomes unstuck, and say, *How could I have known?*

Use this practice whenever an unknown regret shows up, to shift your attention to grief and the need to grieve.

REGRETS THAT ARE KNOWN BUT UNINTENDED

At sixteen, sitting in that unkind gynecologist's office, I was scolded for not menstruating and restricting food. His words were brutal—not just because they were cruel, but because I knew on some level he was right. My behavior was harming my body and I regretted it. This is an example of a known regret. But even as I blamed myself, I knew if I could have changed, I would have. I just didn't know how. I wasn't intentionally harming my body, as the gynecologist suggested. Did I regret what was happening? Of course I did. Did I mean to do it? No, I did not.

Some regrets stem from clearly knowing that something you have done or are currently doing is causing harm to your body. Behaviors that have been unkind to your body, ignoring your body's ongoing messages of pain and discomfort, and any behaviors that have led your body away from its natural balance and homeostasis will, over time, produce these regrets.

You may be wondering, "If I'm self-harming or body-harming, isn't that intentional?" No, it is not. No one is born wanting to harm themselves. Our bodies are designed for protection—they desire to feel safe. Self-harm and body-harm arise when we lose our sense of safety, often for reasons we don't fully understand (many of which you learned about in part one). If you are self-harming, you are trying to make yourself feel safe, but when you engage in behaviors that harm your body, you are not acting from a grounded place or exercising your agency.

I knew restriction wasn't what my body needed, but I didn't know another way to feel safe. Similarly, Amelia, a study participant, reported, "I didn't give myself diabetes, but I know I didn't support my body from getting it either." Known regrets come from choices made in dysregulated states, often when the grief underneath feels unbearable. These regrets often bring self-criticism: "How could you do that?" or "You know better!" Bring mindful attention to these thoughts and respond with self-compassion: *Yes, I know, but I don't (or didn't) mean to do it. There was so much happening I had yet to understand.*

Take a moment to pause here. Gently sway or gently rock your body. Facing the reality that we may have caused harm is hard, but self-compassion is fierce and strong and unafraid to meet these moments.

The Known but Unintended Regrets

1. Please take this moment to reflect on the known but unintended regrets that your body has experienced from your past and present actions.

2. List each regret, and after each one, write the words, *Yes, I know what I did or didn't do, but I didn't mean to do it. There was so much happening I had yet to understand.*

3. Place your hands on your lap, palms up, and move your hands and arms in an upward sweeping motion, lifting toward your belly, heart, throat, and eyes. Let this be a fluid motion. Can you notice grief moving?

4. Sense your breath lifting inward and upward with each sweep upward, as if clearing the space inside, as you say, *Yes, I know, but I didn't mean to do it. There was so much happening I had yet to understand.*

Use this practice whenever a known but unintended regret shows up, to shift your attention to grief and the need to grieve.

MUDDY-WATER REGRETS

Pain, illness, or suffering in our bodies often leaves us confused and wondering if things could have been different. On days when my body suffers—during bouts of inflammation or medication changes—I find my mind wandering into the muddy waters of body regret. I reflect on the past and present, wondering, "Would I have developed an eating disorder or autoimmune illnesses if I hadn't had those exceptional childhood experiences? Did years of restriction harm my endocrine system? If I hadn't grown up in an alcoholic household, would my body be healthier?" Maybe. Maybe not.

Muddy-water regrets are about asking questions about things that typically have no answers. They arise as we try to connect our past to our present physical state. Sometimes the cause-and-effect is clear, but often it's not. Even when we have answers, we still need to grieve—knowing why something is the way it is doesn't take away the pain. For example, a client with a high A1C wondered if her past binge eating behaviors caused her high blood sugar levels. Another, who had recently been diagnosed with breast cancer, wondered if all the exceptional experiences she had as a child contributed to its development and if starting therapy sooner could have prevented it.

You may not have a clear answer as to why your body is struggling. It might or might not be related to past events. This uncertainty can be a challenging situation for our minds to grasp. Remember, our minds seek clear answers, but often clarity doesn't exist in these muddy waters. What does exist and is waiting to be attended to is grief, which, if left unattended, often turns into fear. Fear pushes you back into the endless search for the newest promise of a cure or the latest diet. We can't be certain if any of these will be effective, as only your body truly knows what it needs.

Even if you were to get answers to these questions, they will not help you grieve or build the relationship with your body you long for. If you find yourself lost in this trap, remind yourself it's a normal human response born from uncertainty and unresolved grief.

Instead of staying stuck in the loop of questioning, try to acknowledge this grief. Name it, come down to the ground, and gently soothe it so you can shift into grieving and return to your center.

The Muddy-Water Regrets

- Reflect on the muddy-water regrets your body has experienced that leave you wondering about the past causes of present pain, illness, or suffering.

- List each regret, and after each one, write the words, *This may be the reason or it may not be.*

- Place your hands on your lap, palms up, and move your hands and arms in an upward sweeping motion, lifting toward your belly, heart, throat, and eyes. Let this be a fluid motion. Can you notice grief moving?

- Sense your breath lifting inward and upward with each sweep upward, as if clearing the space inside, saying, *This may be related, or it may not be.*

Muddy-water regrets are complex, but clarity can emerge from this complexity. Just as the lotus blooms in muddy waters, you can find a new way to cope with confusing regrets. Like all regrets, these require grieving—perhaps even more so, because they often stem from current suffering. Your desire to understand and help your body is a sign that your capacity for self-compassion and your relationship with your body are growing. Pause and gently rock or sway as you acknowledge, *I am just trying to understand and help.*

Shame, Safety, and Self-Compassion

The word *shame* evokes a strong response in most women. Notice what happens inside as you read the word. Study participants described the sensation of shame in their bodies as darkness, thick glue, fear and torment, a false self, turning away and against, silent, lurking, avoidance, and dissociation. Shame also disguises grief and the need to grieve.

Shame arises when we see our bodies as problematic in the eyes of the world. Like diet-culture messages, shame can become absorbed in our bodies. The author and activist Sonya Renee Taylor calls out diet culture as a system that profits off of our body shame.[3] Shame develops young, but it's not a natural response toward our bodies— no one is born feeling shame toward themselves or their body. The self-compassion expert Chris Germer calls shame an innocent emotion that all humans experience.[4] It's important to remember that shame is young and innocent at its core, arising from our desire to be loved and cared for.

Shame is often experienced as a profound attack on our sense of self, affecting our sense of safety and protection and throwing us off-center. When shame is present, your autonomic nervous system perceives it as a threat, making you feel vulnerable, unsafe, and unprotected. During moments of shame, self-critical thoughts intensify, fueling a negative cycle. The good news: Self-compassion is the antidote. It soothes shame and helps restore balance. Grieving is not scary to your body—it's natural. Shame, on the other hand, feels unsafe. Each time you interrupt shame and allow yourself to grieve, you reinforce self-compassion.

Meeting Shame with Self-Compassion

This practice is available as an audio recording at www.shambhala.com/body-forgiveness-practices. It will help you locate and describe shame in your body and soothe it with self-compassion.

1. Sit comfortably. Close your eyes or keep a soft gaze. Take a few release breaths in through your nose and out through your mouth.

2. Reflect on the word *shame* and notice any shifts inside. If your mind pulls away, gently return by swaying or rocking and finding your center.

3. Remembering back to the Your Body as a Canvas practice, sense where you would paint shame inside your body. Where do you feel it trapped or glued?

4. Place a hand, blanket, or pillow on this area. Feel the softness and gentle pressure.

5. Acknowledge: *This is shame. I see you and I feel you. My body was not born with this.*

6. Circle the edge of shame with your hand, staying at a comfortable distance, not too close or too far. Send soothing energy, such as the warmth of your hand or imagine warm water gently dripping into the space where shame feels held, to break up the stuckness.

7. Approach shame with the balanced energy of intention to stay present and soothe it. Take some release breaths.

8. Repeat: *This is shame. I see you and I feel you, and I can soothe you.*

9. Imagine how young this part of you is. Your innocent self and
    your body never asked for shame—they only wanted to feel
    safe, protected, and loved.

Notice what's happening inside you. Has something shifted? If so, in
what way? Has shame loosened its grip? Has grief come to the surface? If so, embrace it. Wrap your arms around your body and sway
and rock. When you're ready, sweep your arms upward from belly
to heart, throat, and eyes. This helps transform grief over shame
into true grieving.

Taking Care of Your Needs

My body has never felt the same since being diagnosed with Graves'
disease and thyroid removal. Synthetic hormones don't fully replace
what my body lost, and inflammation is a daily challenge. It took
years to adjust, regain balance, and return to a state of homeostasis.
It also took years to move grief into grieving. As a trauma therapist, I
know how exceptional experiences—especially in childhood—affect
our autonomic functioning and ability to maintain balance. Our bodies register trauma, and ongoing experiences can impact our health.
Gabor Maté, in *When the Body Says No: Exploring the Stress-Disease
Connection*, reveals that 80 percent of autoimmune diseases occur
in women. According to Maté, there are common traits among those
who develop such conditions, including enduring exceptional experiences in early childhood and learning to dismiss their emotions
and bodily sensations in favor of caring for others.[5] When we prioritize other people's needs over our own, when we are caregivers for
others at our own expense, there is a cost.

Rose Hackman, in *Emotional Labor*, describes how women are
socialized to take on the burden of emotional labor, both in the
workplace and at home. We are socialized to believe we are better

at the role of caregiver and empathizer than are men, despite findings that show little to no difference between the genders when it comes to empathy and compassion toward others. Emotional labor refers to the mental effort involved in handling the everyday tasks needed to maintain relationships and keep a household or process running smoothly. This work often goes unrecognized and is typically carried out more by women, who silently shoulder this unappreciated burden.[6]

Women and girls tend to adopt these enculturated gender norms at very young ages, and the caregiver role tends to follow them across their life spans. According to public-health studies, women aged forty-five and older provide the majority of care to their family members and friends, including informal care, and they juggle multiple roles while caregiving, such as hands-on health provider, care manager, friend, companion, surrogate decision-maker, and advocate.[7] That's a lot of need! Let's pause for a moment to reflect on what happens to you and your body's needs in the process of caring for others.

Your Needs Over My Own

Women are often conditioned to put others' needs first. This can become so ingrained that it may feel like a natural instinct, but all bodies—regardless of gender, race, size, or ability—deserve care, love, and attention. That includes having your needs met equally with others. This reflection invites you to consider how you have met your body's needs. Reflect on and journal about these questions:

- What is your earliest memory of caring for another's needs?

- What is your earliest memory of feeling responsible for another's needs?

- Is it easier to recognize and attend to others' needs over your own? How does this show up? Do you forget to feed yourself but not your pets or children? Do you allow your children to nap, but not yourself?

- Is it easy to forfeit what your body needs to care for someone else?

- What's it like inside when you consider taking care of your own needs first?

Reflect on these often, especially the last one. Does it throw you off-center? Does it produce shame or feel unnatural? If so, you're not alone. Like many women, I was raised to believe that focusing on myself meant neglecting others. This belief was a form of grief I had to confront. At first prioritizing your own needs may feel uncomfortable and bring up grief. But you've learned how to shift grief, and over time it gets easier. Prioritizing your needs is compassionate. Studies show that when we care for our own suffering, we're better able to care for others.[8] It doesn't have to be "my needs or theirs"—it can be both. Compassion teaches us, "May I give this to myself so I can give to another."

Grief and Food Are Intimately Connected

As a teen with anorexia, one of the foods I restricted for years was pizza. Pizza has a significant history for me—it was my favorite food and a symbol of connection with my father, who owned an Italian restaurant. I learned to make everything from dough to sauce and even how to toss the dough. After his passing, I didn't realize that grief was why my feelings about pizza shifted from love to pain.

During this vulnerable time, the diet culture's messages that it was bad to consume carbs and fat made it easier to focus on the food than on the grief. Eventually I allowed pizza back into my life after acknowledging and processing the grief. Years later, when I was diagnosed with celiac disease, I had to give up pizza again, but this time for my body's health. Interestingly, I started dreaming about pizza, pasta, and bread—the very foods I'd once restricted out of grief were now the ones I needed to mourn and let go of again. My grief was not just about missing these foods, it was about missing the love, joy, and connection they represented.

As you learned in part one, your relationship with food began with love, joy, and connection—free from regret, shame, or suffering. There was a time when food was simply nurturing and compassionate. If this has changed for you, know it was never your fault. We're all born with an innocent, natural relationship with food, and with the ability to listen to our body's cues and respond accordingly. If you still have this connection, appreciate it, as it's not always easy to maintain.

For many women, this relationship was disrupted long ago by someone or something that interrupted the communication. If you find yourself here, know you never intended for your relationship with food to change, nor did your body. You never meant to demonize foods, lose your connection to your body, or let your mind dictate your needs. You never meant to suppress the fond memories or lose agency around food. You and your body are mourning the relationship with food and all that's been lost.

EMBODIED REFLECTION AND PRACTICE

Grieving Food

1. How long has it been since you had a natural relationship with food, one that feels unburdened, safe, and protective?

2. What messages took this innocent relationship away?

3. What beliefs have you held about certain foods for so long?

4. What foods have been absent from your life that once brought you and your body love and connection? (Consider family recipes and foods unique to your ethnicity.)

5. Pause and place your hands on your lap, palms up, and sweep your arms upward toward your belly, heart, throat, and eyes. Let the movement be fluid.

6. Sense your breath lifting inward and upward with each sweep upward, clearing space inside, and say the words, *So much has been lost. My body and I never wanted it to be this way.*

By now you may realize there's no way to avoid grief. Deception tries to mask it with blame. Regret covers it with "would've, should've, could've." Shame tries to convince you something is wrong with you, your body, or your relationship with food. This cycle can trap you. Ultimately, what you're facing is grief and the need to grieve. These moments are your body's way of communicating all the years of unmet needs and self-sacrifice, the longing to be at peace with yourself and in the world. Pause and be present in these moments. Allow self-compassion to emerge. Feel the grief and shift into grieving. In the next chapter you will learn how body forgiveness helps to hold and soften grief as it is expressed. For now, feel the heaviness. Come down to the ground, rest, and be held.

Make room for the darkness. Don't be afraid of the grief.
—JOSEPHINE, A STUDY PARTICIPANT

7

EMBODYING FORGIVENESS
It's Not What You Think

> Learning to forgive takes time, sometimes years. So be
> patient as you weave a little forgiveness into your daily
> routine as a way of strengthening your capacity to forgive.[1]
> —MARK COLEMAN

THE SEVENTH STAGE of body forgiveness is about embodying forgiveness and discovering how it feels within your body. This chapter introduces the concept of body forgiveness and offers a new, deeper understanding of what forgiveness means. If the idea of forgiveness feels hard to relate to in the context of your body, that's perfectly okay. As you'll see, body forgiveness may not be what you expect. It has little to do with your thoughts and everything to do with what you sense and feel. You'll soon learn the felt difference between forgiving from the mind and forgiving from the heart-mind, which is what body forgiveness is about. When forgiveness is centered in the heart, it creates a release and relief in your body that you can feel right away.

> It's not about doing something wrong. You have to think
> about forgiveness in a different way. It's not an apology;
> it's an understanding.
> —MARTHA, STUDY PARTICIPANT

How We Usually Define Forgiveness

Reflect on the word *forgiveness*. What do you notice inside as you sit with it? How do you feel about the idea of forgiving your body? Pay attention to your immediate experience, both in your mind and body. Do you feel resistance? Do thoughts rush in about all the wrongdoings you've done to your body, or that your body has done to you? Do you feel thrown off-center or notice tightness or a quickening heartbeat?

If the idea of forgiving your body feels challenging, there are many reasons for this, none of which are your fault. They stem from disembodiment and the sense of disconnection from your body. When you see your body as separate from your mind, it's easy to blame it for not looking, cooperating, or behaving as you wish. This disconnect can make the concept of forgiveness toward your body hard to grasp.

Many people find it easier to forgive others for their wrongdoings than to forgive themselves or their bodies. Forgiveness often feels like a struggle, dependent on whether your body performs as you want or meets your expectations. Some people can intellectually grasp forgiveness but struggle to feel it physically. Unfortunately, trying to forgive your body from the mind is often unsuccessful.

Why Forgiving from the Mind Doesn't Work

I first noticed the difference between mind forgiveness and body forgiveness eight years ago while teaching my first Befriending Your Body Program for people struggling with disordered eating and body image. During a forgiveness practice, I saw how challenging it was for participants. They felt blocked and off-center as thoughts of the past flooded in, bringing with it anger, resentment, disgust, and loathing. Most spiraled back into feeling betrayed by their bodies. Statements like "I'm not ready to forgive myself" and "Why should I forgive my body? It has caused me so much distress" were common.

Forgiveness felt impossible for these women to imagine. I could feel the heaviness in the group, and I related to them—I had once felt the same way. Trying to forgive yourself from your mind spirals you into the past, leaving you with shame and the belief that you need to exonerate all the wrongs you think you've committed toward your body. It throws you off your center and makes it hard to be present to what you need now to heal. This barrier to forgiveness grows after years of unaddressed grief and disconnection from your body. Trying to approach forgiveness solely through the mind can lead to more struggle and further disconnection.

Remember, as you learned in chapter 6, you don't need to exonerate yourself. You never intended to harm your body. While you may wish some behaviors or disconnection had never happened, there are complex reasons for the development of those behaviors. No one is born wanting to harm their body; you did not come into this world with these behaviors or this lack of relationship. Now is a good time to remind yourself of the compassionate words from chapter 5: *I never asked for this.* You never asked to feel disembodied or to lose this vital connection.

Let's pause and practice with the compassionate phrases from chapter 2, to remind yourself how disembodiment developed:

- *May I now understand what my body has endured in this world, including the messages it has received, the beliefs it has held, and the judgments and shame it has experienced.*

- *May I come to understand that because of these messages, it was easy to separate from, dislike, belittle, judge, and be unkind to my body.*

- *Through this understanding, may I ignite the commitment to heal, balance, and repair this relationship. May I come to understand that I never asked for it to be this way.*

Practice these statements whenever you find yourself stuck in the loop of trying to forgive from your mind. Understanding why you lost your way with your body helps you face regrets and grief, allowing forgiveness to open.

Making Amends with Your Body

When you allow yourself to confront the pain and grief associated with your body, you move toward what the researcher Frederic Luskin calls "intrapersonal forgiveness," the act of forgiving yourself in relationship to your body.[2] It involves intentionally facing feelings and regrets with compassion, including acknowledging the actions and behaviors that harmed your body. This is a crucial step toward body forgiveness and a better relationship with your body.

To begin, ask yourself: *If my body could speak, what would it say about the actions or behaviors I regret?* While it may feel unusual to approach your body this way, it's similar to practicing forgiveness in any important relationship. Joyce, a study participant, said, "I had to ask forgiveness from my body for the ways I harmed it. I had to reflect on what I have done and what I am doing now." JG shared, "I had to ask my body to forgive me. I am sorry for shutting you down."

EMBODIED REFLECTION

Asking Your Body for Forgiveness

What would you ask your body to forgive you for? Remember, your body's nature is compassion and forgiveness. It will not judge or criticize you. If judgment or shame arises as you reflect on this question, pause, place a hand or two on your heart, and gently sway or rock to remind yourself that your body is always willing to listen and receive your attention.

Maybe you wish to ask forgiveness for past or current behaviors, body judgments or criticisms, ignoring your body's signals, or lack of care. You could use these words: *Dear body, I am sorry if I caused you any harm. My actions were unintentional. There was a lot I needed to learn. Can you forgive me? I did the best I could at that time.*

Forgiveness Is a Continuous Cycle

Asking for forgiveness from your body is a courageous act that involves confronting past regrets and admitting that you may have let your body down before—while recognizing that you may disappoint it in the future. Remember, your body is forgiving by nature. If it could speak, it would forgive you. Practicing intrapersonal forgiveness requires acknowledging that this process is ongoing, and there will be times you let your body down again, just as your body may let you down.

In a romantic relationship, forgiveness often includes a commitment to do your best to avoid further harm. But your relationship with your body is more complex than most love relationships. You can't guarantee you'll never dislike your body again or act unkindly toward it—and your body can't make promises either. No matter how well you care for it, your body will get sick, age, and change over time. Sometimes it won't function as you wish, and it will eventually lose some abilities.

Disappointment between you and your body is inevitable. Because of this, forgiveness isn't a one-time event—it's an ongoing process, something to practice daily, even multiple times a day. It's a lifelong journey. Lisa, a study participant, said, "Forgiveness is a continual, ongoing process. It's a practice because there will always be something to forgive." Joan, a study participant, said she is trying to weave a little forgiveness in each day: "Like a basket, me and my body."

Since there will always be challenges, you may find yourself pulling away from your body, feeling annoyed, angry, or frustrated. These feelings are signaling a moment of grief. As the study participant Willow said, "When there is guilt or grief, there is an opportunity to turn the knob that brings forgiveness back into your life."

It's not the moments of being pulled away that matter most; it's how you come back and learn to stay present in your body when forgiveness is needed.

EMBODIED PRACTICE

Staying with Your Body

This practice is available as an audio recording at www.shambhala .com/body-forgiveness-practices. It will help you remain present in your body during difficult times. It reconnects you by tuning into your body's internal awareness, especially in areas holding tension from body criticism or unkindness. Noticing and naming these sensations helps you stay with them, allowing somatic release and cultivating compassion and forgiveness.

1. Sit comfortably and gently move your head side to side, up and down.

2. Massage the sides and back of your neck with your hands. What do you notice beneath your fingers? Describe the texture and quality of the tissue. The more you can describe the sensations, the more you get to know your body.

3. Find one area to focus on—maybe a spot of tension stands out.

4. Cover the area with your hand. Notice the temperature and pressure of your hand meeting this area.

5. Close your eyes. Soften any critical or self-blaming thoughts. Say, *May I just be with this sensation*, and focus your attention on the space beneath your hand.

6. Get to know the sensation—the particular characteristics of the tension and holding in this spot. Be as descriptive as possible. Notice if it changes at all as you attend to it. Is it ready to soften?

7. Stay with the sensation, without blame or shame, comforting it through your touch. Say, *I am here now. I'm not going anywhere.*

It's common to have moments of relief and connection with your body, and it's also common to leave your body again and feel angry at it or disconnected from it. Building moments of relief and learning to stay with them is one way to make forgiving yourself and your body a regular practice.

Softening and Letting Go

Body forgiveness means embracing a new understanding of forgiveness—one that goes beyond rigid ideas of right and wrong. Unlike forgiveness from the mind, body forgiveness is a heart-mind experience that you feel, not just think about. When you forgive from the heart, an internal softening and letting go begins. You may have felt this softening in the last practice.

Softening starts by reminding yourself that the fractured relationship you feel with your body isn't your fault. It developed in a disconnected, disembodied culture, shaped by systems that pull you away from your body. Softening allows you to be present and soothes the grief and hope that still longs for a different past. Here is how some of the study participants described softening into forgiveness:

"I had to let go of everything that interfered with forgiveness. My body was begging to awaken and to breathe. I couldn't breathe. I collapsed and was raw with a body that couldn't work. I had no choice (but to forgive) and rebuild."—WILLOW

"I cry a lot. That releases the tightness and keeps my compassionate connection going, the 'we.'"—SARAH

"Letting go of the vigilance is forgiveness."—AMELIA

"You can't think about letting go—you have to let go through the body: move, shake, swim. It's happening all the time; something inside moves and shifts."—SOPHIA

"Letting go is humongous! My mind needs to let go, and my body can help facilitate that."—PEARL

Letting go of hope for a different past can be hard. Grief doesn't simply fade away. Your body can't erase the pain it may have caused you over the years, nor can you erase the pain you believe you've inflicted on your body. You and your body can't escape the pain you might still encounter in the world. Instead, you and your body must grieve and soften together.

EMBODIED PRACTICE

What Letting Go Feels Like

Letting go in your body means feeling a release, but you can't know what release feels like until you experience it in your body. I encourage you to lie down for this practice—on the floor or in bed. Once the movements become familiar, you can practice them sitting or standing any time during your day.

- Lie on your back with arms in a T position and legs open wider than your hips.

- Practice release breathing: Inhale through your nose, exhale through your mouth. On the exhale, open your mouth wide and stick out your tongue—in yoga, this is called Lion's Breath. Take three to five complete breaths, making your exhale more audible each time.

- Begin to move your feet in a windshield-wiper motion—toward each other, then outward. Start slow, then quicken the pace. Slow down and pause to notice the movement in your feet and legs, even in stillness.

- Shake your feet and let the motion travel up your legs, eventually allowing your whole leg to join in. Slow down and pause to notice the movement in your feet, legs, and elsewhere, even in stillness.

- Move your hands from palms up to palms down. Notice how moving your hands moves your arms and even your shoulders. Start slow, then quicken the pace, building up to a speed that feels natural to your body. Slow down and pause to notice movement in your hands and arms, even in stillness.

- Shake your hands and let the motion travel up your arms, allowing your whole arm to join in. Slow down and pause to notice movement in your hands, arms, and shoulders, even in stillness.

- Gently turn your head side to side a few times. Then nod your head in a "yes" motion. Move slowly and gently. Pause and come to silliness, noticing how even gentle movements can release something inside.

- Tap your fingertips from the back of your head to the sides, then to your forehead, above your brows, and down your jawline. Start slow, then quicken the pace. Slow down and pause to notice the movement in your head, face, and jaw, even in stillness.

You don't have to know what your body is letting go of. You don't have to analyze it. Just feel it happening. That's the beauty of this kind of letting go. As Amelia said, there's no vigilance behind it.

Mindfully Letting Go

The Buddhist teacher Jack Kornfield explains that letting go in the mind doesn't mean eliminating or discarding something—it means allowing thoughts to simply exist.[3] Just as letting go in the body is a softening and release, letting go in the mind is an easing and allowing. This shift happens as you move from trying to change or suppress thoughts to permitting them to be. My study participants shared:

> "I had to let go of the way I think, like, 'Oh, it'll be when . . .' I'm letting go of trying to make things happen in a certain way. Fear does not have to drive my behavior. It's all part of forgiveness as it lets new ideas in."—MARTHA

> "I had to let go of the 'coulds, woulds, and shoulds,' along with the 'if onlys.'"—JOYCE

> "My body is going through its own changes whether I want it to or not. I had to let go and surrender to it. It's like a remembrance to join."—REBECCA

As you learned in chapter 5, mindfulness means focusing attention on the present moment with kindness. Mindfully letting go means noticing thoughts that distract you from your body without judgment and allowing them to pass. These thoughts will arise—it's natural. The challenge is to notice when these thoughts appear and meet them with compassion. As Rebecca said, remember to join your body rather than getting pulled away into disembodiment.

Allowing Thoughts to Be

1. Take a release breath by inhaling through your nose and exhaling through your mouth. Call to mind your last would've, could've, or should've thought. Notice how it shifts you away from your center. Shake out your legs and arms, then come back to meet this thought in a new way.

2. Place your hands on your heart or another soothing spot. Repeat: *My body and I did the best we could do. We did the best we could do. I'm joining with my body rather than against it.*

3. Take another release breath. Call to mind your last fearful thought about your body—maybe about its ability, health, function, or size. Notice how just recalling this thought shifts you away from your center. Shake out your legs and arms, then come back to meet this thought in a new way.

4. Place your hands on your heart or another soothing spot. Repeat: *This is fear. My body and I can meet this fearful thought without reactivity. We can meet this together. I'm joining with my body rather than against my body.*

These thoughts will come up again and again. When you meet them and allow them to be, they may not disappear, but they will fade into the background, letting you rejoin your body. Each time you do, forgiveness takes place and allows new thoughts and ideas to unfold.

Forgiveness quiets the mind and lets you listen to
the voice of your body first.
—Willow, study participant

The Deeper Understanding That Your Body Never Meant You Any Harm

Forgiveness from the heart recognizes that your body never intended to cause you pain or suffering. It never meant to deceive you, betray you, or leave you feeling alone. Your body never wanted to change, become sick, age, or stand out—it longed to fit in. It never wanted to scare you or make you feel unsafe, or to be teased, hated, or harmed. Your body longs for the same things your mind and heart do: freedom from suffering, stability, safety, and connection. It seeks the same steadiness and peace you long for.

Notice what's happening inside you right now. Even a small glimmer of internal change—tension releasing, tears forming, or the river of emotion moving differently—signals a softening within. Pause and be with the felt sense of this shift toward your body. This is body forgiveness.

Your Body Didn't Ask for This Either

Until now, you may have embraced the idea, "I never asked for this." But have you considered that your body never asked for harm or suffering either? This perspective is essential for developing a subjective and relational understanding of your body—one that honors it as a living, feeling, sensing part of you.

This viewpoint respects both your experiences and your body's experiences. It acknowledges the painful memories you and your body recall. While you have wanted many things from your body, your body also has wants and needs from you. Understanding your body's experiences through this lens is another step toward embodiment.

In chapter 4 you learned how messages from the world, combined with your life experiences, complicated your relationship with your body and left you believing you were in an unsafe body. Your body, meanwhile, was just doing what bodies do—trying to find its way back to safety. Each exceptional experience leaves your internal system searching for balance. After a stressful event, it typically takes your body twenty to sixty minutes to regain homeostasis. Consider that for just one event. Now imagine what happens when multiple stressors and exceptional experiences are happening at the same time. Your body has endured a lot.

Pause, place your hands somewhere on your body that brings softening and comfort, and acknowledge that you have held a lot—and your body has held a lot for you. Say this to your body: *I know you have held a lot for me. Thank you for holding all of this for me.*

Avoiding the Second Arrow

Even uncomfortable sensations—like intense anxiety or a sense of being shut down—are your body's way of trying to protect you. Learning to respond differently in moments that feel unsafe can help your body regain peace.

A Buddhist teaching about the second arrow explains how your reactions during suffering can either ease or worsen your pain. Imagine you're having a neutral day with your body image until someone comments on your size or food choices. That comment might push you off-center, especially if you've felt vulnerable to such remarks for years. The first arrow that brings suffering to you and your body is the initial comment, which lands as hurtful, followed closely by your body's reaction. Your body remembers this threat, and your nervous system, sensing danger, rushes in to protect you by activating the stress response system, flooding your body with stress hormones and increasing tension throughout. The second arrow is the self-critical thoughts and feelings you have about your body, along with frustration and judgment of how your mind or body has reacted. Your body may continue this protective response until you learn to meet it in a new way.

Noticing What Your Body Holds for You

This practice helps you meet moments of body suffering in a new way.

- Recall your last moment of challenge in your body that produced uncomfortable sensations.

- What did you notice? Was there a shift in your energy into over- or underdrive? What sensations did you notice? Are you experiencing any of these sensations now?

- Is this body reaction familiar? If so, how long has your body responded this way?

- Meet this moment with understanding: *You have held moments like this for me for so long.*

- Place your hands somewhere on your body that feels safe and soothing.

- Gently move your body and repeat: *I'm so sorry you had to hold this for so long.*

- Pause and notice any softening inside or any change in the flow of your river of emotion. This is body forgiveness taking place.

This practice helps your body feel seen and supported—and regain balance more quickly after a stressful event.

What If Your Body Isn't Ready to Let Go?

Sometimes your mind is ready to let go, but your body isn't. As a child I experienced significant social anxiety—my body reacted with a racing heart, sweating, a quiet voice, and a strong urge to hide. Teachers failed to recognize my struggles, and instead of compassion, I faced ridicule and criticism, which led me to shame, blame, and get angry at my body for its reactions—a perfect example of the second arrow.

This social anxiety continued into adulthood. My work now involves teaching and lecturing to large groups, and I wish my body had released its sense of unsafety. It hasn't. For years, I struggled with anger and frustration at my body's responses. Then one day I stopped, placed my hands on my racing heart, and paused. My body was still reacting as if I were that six-year-old. I pressed my hands into my chest more firmly and felt their warmth at my heart.

In that moment I felt sadness for my body. While my mind was ready to let go of the past, my body wasn't. It needed more time to process past experiences. It needed patience, compassion, and understanding. As my mind softened, tears flowed and I experienced forgiveness toward my body. I forgave it for not being ready yet. I accepted that this was just how it was for my body in that moment.

It Is Just How It Is for My Body

The following reflection will help you build a deeper understanding of and respect for your body's release process.

- Consider a reaction your body has had for a long time—maybe a feeling or sensation that's hard to shake, even though you say you are over it or done with it.

- What do you notice about this experience inside? How would you describe it? Does it happen in specific situations?

- How have you tried to cope?

- Call the experience to mind now. Sometimes even recalling these experiences will evoke the feeling or sensations again.

- Place your hands somewhere on your body that feels safe and soothing.

- Close your eyes and let the pressure of your hands acknowledge your presence. Pause and breathe.

- Acknowledge the following to yourself:

My mind wants this experience to shift, but I understand my body may not be ready to release this yet.

My mind wants this to go away and be left in the past, but my body is still figuring it out.

My body may need more time.

May I offer patience, understanding, and forgiveness to my body for not being ready yet.

May I trust in my body's wisdom to release this and trust in its safety as it is ready.

For now, this is just how it is for my body.

This practice reminds you that while your mind may be ready to move on, your body may not be. Your body has carried so much for a long time. When your body has been conditioned to move away from its center, it takes time to feel safe again. As you acknowledge your body's reactions and respond with patience, understanding, and compassion, your body will gradually learn that it's safe to release its protective armor. Trust that your body knows when it's ready to heal; it just needs support along the way.

Attending to Your Body's Needs

One of the most complex concepts in embodiment is the difference between what your mind wants for your body and what your body actually needs—the needs of the mind versus the needs of the body.

We are born embodied with only body needs. Consider a baby in a wet diaper: It feels discomfort, recognizes distress, and has a need—for a diaper change. As you grow and your thinking brain develops, you move away from knowing what your body needs. Your mind's ideas override your body's messages, and you stop listening and responding to your body's needs. Still, your body continues to communicate through overt and subtle sensory cues. Every time you register a sensation, your body is requesting a response.

Listening and responding to your body's requests can be challenging. Most of us are taught to ignore our body's signals and to turn away from basic needs like rest, nourishment, safety, and connection. The attention that your body's early needs received influences your ability to recognize and respond to those needs later in life. If you find it difficult to tune in to your body's sensations and needs, you're not alone. The good news is you can relearn—starting by acknowledging your body's needs throughout the day.

Attuning to Your Body's Needs

Use these questions as a guide throughout the day to pause, slow down, attune, and attend to your body's needs, or as a journal prompt at the end of the day.

- **PROPER REST:** Resting your body takes many forms. Rest can mean a nap, slowing the pace of your walk, pausing to stretch, resting your head, closing your eyes for a few seconds, or curling up on the couch in a soft blanket at the end of the day. Ask yourself: *Was I able to attend to my body's need for rest today? If not, what pulled me away?*

- **PROPER NOURISHMENT:** Proper nourishment is an essential need of your body, and it can take many forms. This includes eating with regularity and consistency throughout the day, not skipping meals, and paying attention to the amounts and types of foods you choose. Your body deserves to feel satiated and satisfied at each meal, and it benefits from variety in textures, tastes, colors, and even food temperatures. Ask yourself: *Was I able to attend to my body's need for nourishment today? If not, what pulled me away?*

- **FEELING SAFE AND CONNECTED:** Another way to describe feeling safe is being in your center. It is unrealistic to expect to feel this way all the time, but you can look for the moments when you return to safety. When you do, you'll naturally feel more connected with your body. You can support your body in returning to these moments throughout the day by paying attention to your autonomic functioning (see chapter 4)—specifically by noticing what's happening inside your body, in your environment, and in your interactions with others. Ask yourself: *Was I able to attend to my body's fluctuating internal states and need for safety today? If not, what pulled me away?*

Reflect on these categories daily to continue to increase your capacity to recognize your body's needs and build awareness around areas that may require more attention and care from you.

This chapter offers a new understanding of body forgiveness—one that finally allows you to release the long-held belief that you did something wrong that led to this divide between you and your body. It's finally time to embrace the release and relief in your body and mind that body forgiveness offers. Feel the relief in your mind and embrace the release in your body—your body has been waiting to feel this from you for a long time. Trust that every time you feel an internal shift into softening, you are forgiving your body and yourself. This rejoining is the healing path back home to embodiment. Now that you are here, you will learn all about what it takes to sustain this reconnection through the practice of body forgiveness.

> Every time you find yourself at home in your body again,
> let it be a moment of appreciation and celebration.[4]
> —KATE JOHNSON

Embracing

how do you begin to let go
and trust yourself enough
to lead the way to fields
of wildflowers
to the steps of a house
built just for you
to open the door
and welcome you home
—ZÖE LAWRIE

WELCOME TO PART THREE. Take a moment to appreciate how far you've come in building your relationship with your body. You've made significant progress, and part two provided essential building blocks for this journey. You learned that self-compassion and mindful attention are crucial for gently addressing grief and regret, allowing the process of grieving to unfold. You also discovered a new perspective on forgiveness—what body forgiveness truly means, what it takes to achieve it, and the release and relief it brings. You and your body never meant to harm each other; you've simply been trying to find your way back to each other.

In part three, we address the question: "What comes next?" The answer is, simply, embodiment: learning how to fully arrive, live, sustain, and nurture this newfound relationship. We'll also explore why, to be fair, this journey can still be challenging, and how practicing daily forgiveness toward your body is the answer.

8

EMBRACING PRESENCE

Being Beside Your Body

> Embodied presence is an invitation, again and again, to
> soften, to settle, to relax, to open up to what's here.[1]
> —MARTIN AYLWARD

THE EIGHTH STAGE of body forgiveness is embracing presence. This chapter invites you into a new level of awareness—embodied presence. Merleau-Ponty defines embodied presence as being "beside" your body, a state that arises from attunement and discernment toward your body's physical, emotional, and spiritual needs. Everything you are beginning to understand, sense, and feel contributes to this state. In this chapter you will learn what it feels like to coexist beside your body, how to stay in this presence, and how to meet your body's needs as you grow into this essential next step toward living embodied.

Breath Awareness as a Key to Presence

I've intentionally waited to invite you to practice breath awareness until now. Up to this point, the practices have focused on noticing how your breath changes in response to your nervous system and its shifting states. This was intentional, as focusing on breathing can feel unsafe without a strong foundation of body awareness. Many people feel anxious when they concentrate on their breath and interpret sensations as threatening based on past experiences. For instance, shallow breaths might trigger thoughts or feelings of anxiety. However, you'll come to learn that your breath is an important anchor for remaining connected and present in your body. Staying present to the sensations of your natural breath can lead you back to a centered state and sharpen your ability to rest in the present moment.

Getting to Know Your Natural Breath

This practice helps you discover what it's like to be present with your breath for sensory information and to return to the present moment.

PART ONE

1. You may do this practice sitting or lying down.

2. Take a few release breaths, in through your nose and out through your mouth.

3. Place your hands on your upper chest and notice the movement as you inhale and exhale.

4. Observe the wavelike motion of your chest. Sometimes it moves more, sometimes less. Simply notice this without judgment or trying to figure out why.

5. Be with the movement of this area in response to your breath and say, *This is the way my breath is right now.*

6. Place your hands on your belly, just below your ribcage. Notice the wavelike motion here. Again, just observe without judgment.

7. Be with the movement and say, *This is the way my breath is right now.*

8. Place your hands below your navel. Notice the wavelike motion here. Observe without judgment.

9. Be with the movement and say, *This is the way my breath is right now.*

PART TWO

1. Place your hands on the area where you feel your breath moving the most. Stay here, present to the movement, without forcing your breath or the movement. Let your hands ride the wave of your breath.

2. What happens inside when you remain present with your breath without letting thoughts dictate how it should be?

3. Notice, name, and describe what it's like inside now.

This practice helps you connect with the natural rhythms of your breath, understanding that each breath reflects your body's state in the moment. Rapid breathing during anxiety is just as natural as calm breathing in a centered state. The perception of unnaturalness comes from the mind's judgment. By observing your breath without judgment, you can better receive your body's messages, promoting mindfulness and presence.

Finding Ease in Embodied Presence

Embodied presence is the result of being present—joining with your body and recognizing it as an essential, sensing, feeling part of your identity. This is a subjective, not objective, experience. It's the new relationship you are forming with your body.

Here's an example of embodied presence from my own life, on a morning when I woke up feeling unwell: I placed my hands on my heart and felt my breath. I sensed my energy level to see if my body was ready to wake up, and in what way. That morning my energy was low after a restless night. My body felt heavy and my joints ached. I noticed my mind wandering into "why" questions, but instead of being pulled away, I returned to my body. I focused on the areas that were loudest on a sensory level and noticed inflammation in my joints. I wished it weren't so, and I felt sadness and grief arise. Tears formed. I named this as a moment of grieving.

Then regret came up: "Maybe I wouldn't feel this way if I hadn't eaten what I ate the last few nights." I took a deep breath and came back to my body, naming this as a muddy-water regret. As I returned to being beside my body, I asked what it needed. It wanted to move. I gently moved my achy joints, and the movement felt good. My body wanted more. I got out of bed and onto my yoga mat, letting my joints unwind and release through swaying and rocking. I started to feel more alive as the pain lessened. I eventually stood up, felt my feet on the ground, and did a few balance poses that felt stabilizing. I checked back in—my body felt grounded and strong, my joints unburdened for now. I knew the aches would return, but for that moment my body and I felt free.

When you live from embodied presence, decisions are made with your body in mind, not just from your mind alone. This requires qualities you learned in chapter 5—attention, intention, and balanced energy—but now the approach is softer, gentler, and more natural. Sophia, one of the study participants, described the difference between being present and embodied presence: "Because I have a chronic illness that's painful a lot of the time, I often force myself to be present. But forcing myself all the time isn't necessarily good. Being present feels like I have to gather myself and there's an energy of effort. With embodied presence, there's a lot more ease. It's being naturally who I am, doing my thing, and it's not forced. It just happens on its own without trying. It's those moments when I'm fully at ease. I can feel, this is good, I'm here, I'm not struggling to be here. I'm just there."

As Sophia described, arriving at embodied presence means finding a balance between effort and ease. It involves noticing sensations without forcing awareness. Meg said, "You don't have to be present all the time. You can just create a space to allow that to happen." Think of this space as sitting beside your body, gently turning your attention toward it, and connecting with what it's trying to communicate. It's like a close relationship where no words are needed to understand each other; you begin to rely on feelings and body communication. Insights arise through a less forced, more attentive approach. Rather than trying so hard to figure out what your body needs, you begin to notice and listen to its obvious and now subtle messages.

Being Beside Your Body as You Move

In chapter 3 you explored an embodied reflection called The Way I Move (page 84), becoming more aware of how you inhabit your body throughout the day—in the morning, afternoon, and evening. Now, revisit this reflection through the lens of embodied presence. Imagine turning toward your body and wondering what it may need:

IN THE MORNING: As you wake, pause, turn inward, and notice how quickly your body wants to move from lying down to getting up. Does it want to awaken slowly? How does your body wish to start the day? As you gently turn your attention toward your body, what do you understand about it now?

IN THE AFTERNOON: As your rhythms and energy shift, pause and notice how your body wants to walk or move. Does it want to change pace or stay the same? As you gently turn your attention toward your body, what do you understand about it now?

IN THE EVENING: As the day winds down and you prepare to rest, pause and notice how your body wants to slow down. Has it had the chance to slow its pace? Are there any routines or activities that your body would like to do as it arrives at the end of the day? As you gently turn your attention toward your body, what do you understand about it now?

This reflection helps you find a balance between effort and ease, which is essential for developing body presence. It also helps you recognize when you're shifting into a more intimate connection with your body, allowing you to better understand its current needs rather than being influenced by habitual patterns.

Choosing with Your Body, Not Your Mind

Habitual patterns are behaviors you engage in without much thought or conscious awareness. Over time, these patterns repeat and become mind choices that are often disconnected from sensory awareness. Without guidance from your senses, it's easy to assume what your body wants rather than attune to what it actually needs. Making empowered choices means quieting the habitual mind and imagining that, before each choice, you're essentially meeting your body for the first time—just as when meeting a new person, you wouldn't assume you knew their preferences but would ask. Your body is no different. To assess whether a choice is a body or mind choice, consciously include your body in the decision-making.

By bringing your attention to your body through embodied presence, you can notice patterns that may or may not align with your body's desires. For example, a client realized she habitually did a forty-minute Peloton workout every morning that left her depleted and overly energized, even though her body no longer wanted to rush out of bed. By connecting with embodied presence, she adjusted her routine to ten minutes of gentle stretching and thirty minutes on the Peloton. She started her day feeling more attuned, relaxed, and grounded rather than drained and out of sync.

Body choices arise from tuning into your interoceptive messages and aligning with them in the moment. Reflect on your own patterns around movement and food. Are they body choices or mind choices? Choices influenced by diet culture tend to be based on what you think your body needs, not what your body would choose. External influences—diet culture, family, social circles, and media—can lead you away from empowered choices rooted in your relationship with your body.

Attunement Builds Embodied Presence

The relationship expert Dr. John Gottman defines attunement in romantic relationships as the desire and ability to understand and respect another's inner world.[2] Similarly, attunement to your body means understanding and respecting its inner world, which you've been exploring through interoceptive communication. Like any relationship, your attunement and presence grow as you stay aware and responsive to your body's messages.

Attunement is also about being aware of your desires, wishes, and needs. Just as attunement in relationships fosters connection, respect, and emotional satisfaction, attuning to your body's needs creates the same sense of connection between you and your body. Notice the little things you already do to meet your body's needs, like adjusting your position or choosing comfortable clothing that feels softer, lighter, and freer to your body.

Meeting Your Body for the First Time: Food and Exercise

Reflect on your current food choices. What influences them? Consider all the possible factors—finances, work, home, school, relationships, and roles—that may play a part in what you choose to eat. What might you choose if you weren't guided by external restrictions, habits, or old beliefs? Meet your body for the first time. What does it wish to choose? Does it align with your mind's choices or what you hope to choose?

Reflect on your movement or exercise choices. What influences them? Consider all the possible factors—social pressure, finances, work, health, injury, schedule, relationships, and roles. What would you choose if you weren't guided by external restrictions, habits, or old beliefs? Pause, close your eyes, and imagine what your body truly wishes to do. Meet your body for the first time. What does it wish to choose? Does it align with your mind's choices or what you hope to choose?

Checking in with your body before each choice keeps you aware, attuned, and empowered toward your body's needs.

Allowing Yourself to Receive Pleasure

Attuning to your body's needs also involves exploring pleasure. In chapter 3 we discussed pleasure as the experience of comfort within your body, but it's also about understanding and responding to your desires. Allowing yourself to embrace pleasure in your body is a way to experience and express the fulfillment of your internal desires. This includes enjoying food, engaging in movement that feels good, experiencing soothing touch, and feeling alive and free during moments of sexual arousal. Pleasure is a state of receptivity—being open, aware, willing, and ready to receive. The word *receive* can evoke a strong response. Ask yourself, *Am I ready to receive?* Notice how it makes you feel. Do you experience a sense of contraction or expansion? Many women are conditioned to prioritize giving over receiving, so receiving can be challenging.

If receiving pleasure is hard for you, know that you're not alone. Allowing yourself and your body to receive takes time. Often what prevents us from receiving is the belief that restraint and suppression of bodily desires are valued traits, especially for women. There's a fear that accepting our desires means losing control. The philosopher and feminist theorist Susan Bordo suggests that the mindset of restraint through dieting (withholding food) contributes to the idea that hunger is something dangerous that needs to be controlled.[3] Dr. Niva Piran's research shows that girls learn early to "corset" their sexual desires by striving to appear small, demure, and not too outspoken. They engaged in body alterations, aimed to contain their appetites, and learned early on that they were expected to be "desired yet desire-less," with the understanding that "sexual agency, pleasure, and the freedom to express desire reside with boys."[4]

It's no wonder that receiving pleasure can feel difficult or come with feelings of guilt, shame, or punishment. After each attempt to receive pleasure, check in with yourself—do you feel any contraction or tightness in your body or mind? Are critical, shameful, or regretful thoughts emerging? If so, ensure that your attempt to receive pleasure comes from a place of safety and agency. Even when you feel safe, though, receiving pleasure can be hard, and you're not alone in this discomfort with pleasure. Take a deep breath and place a hand on your body. Recognize how challenging it is as a woman to unwind years of messaging. Connecting with our common humanity in these moments can help you begin to release these messages and return to freely receiving.

Embodying Pleasure

Reflect on the following questions in your journal or an audio note. If it's hard to recall any moments of embodied pleasure, please know you are not alone. Consider the questions based on your present moment from the perspective of "Am I ready to receive?"

- When was the last time you received pleasure from food that aligned with your body's desire? Were you able to remain centered? Were you alone or with others?

- When was the last time you received pleasure from movement that aligned with your body's desire? What was it like inside? Can you describe the sense of pleasure? Were you able to remain centered? Were you alone or with others?

- When was the last time you received pleasure from touch that aligned with your body's desire? What messages did your body give you? Were you able to remain centered? Were you alone or with others?

Embodied Pleasure Creates Alignment Within

Pleasure is inherent to your body's nature. Each time you experience embodied pleasure, your body responds directly and tangibly. Seeking pleasure and avoiding pain are natural instincts. By fulfilling your body's sensory desires, you help restore it to a balanced state.

Experiencing pleasure in moments that feel secure and connected positively impacts your nervous system, leaving you receptive to recognizing and expressing your body's desires. It grounds you and leads to a sense of agency and empowerment. From this state, you can safely navigate between energy states (overdrive and centered), allowing you to be playful, adventurous, and fully engaged in pleasurable experiences. Your body can also transition into a blend of grounded and relaxed (underdrive and centered) energy, enabling you to enjoy touch and sexual pleasure in an empowered, connected way.

How Body Discernment Can Help

Body discernment is the ability to recognize when you're connected to your body's internal, sensory experience. It helps you identify patterns that distract you and pull you away from embodied presence. When connected, you perceive sensory experiences as they are without being sidetracked by judgmental thoughts or intense emotions. This skill requires a level of awareness that enables you to observe what's happening inside while also gently acknowledging thoughts and emotions, then returning to your body. Body discernment involves pausing, reflecting, and reconnecting with your body's sensory awareness.

EMBODIED PRACTICE

Pause, Reflect, and Reconnect: Working with Thoughts and Emotions

This practice is available as an audio recording at www.shambhala.com/body-forgiveness-practices. It will help you build body discernment, notice competing thoughts and emotions, and develop your ability to reconnect to your body.

1. Choose an area of your body that's talking to you—where you notice sensations like tightness or stiffness. If there are many, choose one that's neither too loud nor too quiet. If all seems quiet, choose an area that's stood out to you in the past.

2. Place a hand or fingertips on the area and begin to notice
    and name what it feels like. Provide as much descriptive
    detail as you can.

3. As you notice and describe, say, *I am with my body, and this
    is what I can sense.* Stay with what you notice.

4. If a thought comes in, discern if it's pulling you away from
    or bringing you closer to your body in this moment. Stories,
    judgments, or criticisms tend to pull you away. If this hap-
    pens, gently offer yourself permission for the thoughts to
    quiet so you can pause, reflect, and reconnect to your body.
    When back inside your body, notice if any insight or wisdom
    arises from within. Is there anything your body wishes for
    you to know?

5. Stay with what you notice and be aware of any emotions.

6. If emotions are present, discern if they're pulling you away
    from or bringing you closer to your body in this moment.
    If they pull you away, breathe and gently rock or sway to
    soften the emotion, allowing yourself to pause, reflect, and
    reconnect. When back inside your body, notice if any insight
    or wisdom arises from within. Is there anything your body
    wishes for you to know?

Discerning whether you are truly present with your body—and
whether the thoughts and emotions that arise are part of your
internal experience or are distracting you from it—is essential for
developing embodiment. Be patient with yourself; it's normal to
fluctuate between feeling connected and becoming distracted.
What matters most is using the steps of discernment: Pause, reflect,
and return to your body. It can also help to jot down any repetitive
thoughts or challenging emotions that tend to divert your attention,

so you can recognize them when they arise and more easily return to embodied presence.

The more you practice quieting distracting thoughts and softening emotions, the more you'll realize, as Sophia said, that you don't have to try so hard to be present with your body. You don't have to chase thoughts or emotions away; they can live beside you and your body. Presence isn't perfect awareness—it's a fluid process of moving in and out and back in again.

Embodied Presence as a Transcendent Experience

At its core, embodied presence is a transcendent experience that connects with your body in ways that go beyond the ordinary. Society encourages you to see your body as an image or object, but as you deepen your connection to your body, you move past this limited perspective and embrace the subjective experience of being in your body, focusing instead on developing a new relationship with your body.

Embodied presence is also a state of pleasure. In this state, your mind is light and unburdened by worries, anxiety, or regrets. Moments of true, embodied pleasure—when you and your body are attuned—result in ongoing softening and release. Even after the experience, your body and mind continue to receive it by feeling calm and centered. Moments of embodied presence are special. They allow you to connect deeply to the entirety of an experience, resulting in a sense of connection to all, beyond yourself. This view honors both your body's wisdom and the collective wisdom of generations of women who came before you.

The Body Wisdom of Those Who Came Before You

In chapter 5 you reflected on your body family tree and the messages you absorbed from previous generations. This reflection differs, helping you to view your body beyond the ordinary, and is influenced instead by the *body wisdom* of the many generations of women who came before you who knew what their bodies needed.

Close your eyes and reflect on the women in your lineage who positively influenced you—mothers, sisters, aunts, grandmothers, great-grandmothers. Open your eyes and choose one or several to reflect on: What body wisdom did she pass along? How did she express this? How did her body wisdom influence you? Is it present in your life now? If not, how might you bring it alive again?

For me, I think of my great-aunt Anna. She visited every Sunday, bringing delicious Italian cookies from the Bronx. I loved how tall she stood and how she valued good posture. She cared for herself with food, eating three meals a day and savoring those cookies. I could tell how much pleasure and connection she received from sharing them with us each week. Now, when I stand tall, especially in yogic Mountain Pose, I embody the wisdom of great-aunt Anna. I also allow myself pleasure, especially in connection with others. When I bake and share traditional Italian cookies and desserts, I embody her wisdom.

This reflection helps you connect with the wisdom of the women who inspired you, keeping their presence awake and alive within you.

Touching the Mystery of the Body

Embodied presence also honors the mystery of your body—its history of self-regulation, strength, and health, much of which is beyond your control. The diet and health industry wants you to believe you can influence your body's health and longevity, but we all know there are times you can do everything right and your body will still change, get sick, or feel unwell. If you're fortunate, your body may age peacefully. If you've had health challenges, acknowledge your body's mystery. Every body has its own spiritual and mystical journey and cycle of growth and decline, influenced by your life experiences and of the lives before you. Epigenctics shows that behaviors and environments, both yours and your ancestors', affect how your genes express themselves. Some of these expressions we may be able to influence and some we may not.

Despite all we know, the body remains a profound mystery. This is why we struggle to understand questions like why someone who never exercised might live a long and healthy life while someone else who was an elite athlete experiences illness and death at a young age. My mother passed away from dementia just shy of her ninety-fourth birthday. She never exercised, had a stressful life, often ate unhealthy foods (according to the diet culture), was considered overweight, and had high cholesterol her whole life. Yet her body continued to function and the dementia didn't appear until late in her life. Our bodies are mysterious and have their own unique cycles to fulfill.

Embracing embodied presence means accepting the mystery of your body. What's it like to imagine you're not fully in charge of your body's path? For some, this is freeing; for others, it's unsettling. If it feels scary, pause and return to your center with the practices that have helped you most. When you fully embrace embodied presence, you create space for everything to unfold as it will.

The Still Point Within

This practice helps you rest and feel safe and unburdened within your body. It helps you to drop into a place that can hold whatever your body's path may be.

1. Find a comfortable, supportive seat.

2. Take a few release breaths, inhaling through your nose and exhaling through your mouth.

3. Gently close your eyes or keep a soft gaze. Place one hand on your forehead, gently embracing this area, and let your attention land beneath your hand. Feel the energy from your hand radiate into your forehead, softening and soothing your thoughts. Sense your breath here.

4. Move your hand to your neck, gently embracing this area, and let your attention settle there. Feel the energy from your hand radiate into your neck, softening and soothing your throat. Sense your breath here.

5. Move your hand to your chest, gently embracing this area, and let your attention settle there. Feel the energy from your hand radiate into your chest, softening and soothing your heart. Sense your breath here.

6. Stay here. Deep inside your heart is a still point—a small space untouched by fear and the unknown. This still point can hold and allow your body to be as it is.

7. Imagine what this safe, restful space looks like. Let a color or visual image emerge.

8. Rest here for a while and feel the impact of these words:

In this space I can allow for the mystery of my body
*   to unfold.*
In this space I do not need to control my body.
In this space I can trust my body.
In this space I can be one with my body.

When Body and Spirit Meet

Connecting with your body, feeling safe within, and embracing what brings you joy and freedom allows your spirit to emerge. The meaning of spirit is deeply personal and unique. For some of my study participants, it meant there was no separation between body, mind, and self. Maggie said, "I'm stunned that my body is still here, and I'm awed by that. My body is not something other than me. What's saving my life right now and healing my life is the awareness and experience of the integral body and mind: the unity, inseparability, and integration of what we call body, mind, and spirit." For others, it signified a return to inner bliss or a felt sense of God within that offers protection. Amelia shared, "I'm not sure if it's forgiveness or transcending. Maybe they are both the same. I have a belly but I'm willing to put on a bathing suit because it feels so good to swim. It's my practice. I love the way I move in the pool. It's just a joy. I remember one time being on the beach and I had a swim. I was in such joy . . . it's about meeting my body. When that happens the chatter is gone."

This level of presence—where sensations and emotions merge—allows access to self-transcendent emotions like joy, compassion, and forgiveness, creating a sense of unity between self and body. Ego boundaries weaken, replaced by connection and belonging. From this space your body feels safe to explore and engage in what brings you pleasure and joy, and you remain beside it. In this immersive sensory experience, you and your body become one. Feelings and sensations become fluid, and you are in flow with your body.

This chapter gives you a new way to connect with and honor your body. Embodied presence encourages you to explore your body's needs and desires and allows you and your body to receive the gift of pleasure that you both have been waiting for. Embodied presence helps you appreciate your body's history and spiritual essence every day, and it enables you to embrace the practice of letting go, allowing things to be just as they are.

> What an extraordinary privilege to know that you have within you a refuge that nobody can ever touch. Nobody can take it away from you.[5]
>
> —HELEN TWORKOV

9

EMBRACING BODY EQUANIMITY
Letting Go and Letting Be

If you let go a little, you will have a little peace. If you let
go a lot, you will have a lot of peace. And if you let go
completely, you will have complete peace.[1]
—AJAHN CHAH

THE NINTH STAGE of body forgiveness is embracing letting go. This chapter offers a new perspective on what it means to let go in your body, moment by moment. There's an art to letting go—what I call "body equanimity"—which is part of the later stages of body forgiveness. It's about intentionally releasing and softening in each moment, in your body, mind, and emotions, instead of pushing or straining through the moment. Body equanimity helps you slow down and sustain your attention through challenging sensations, thoughts, and feelings rather than running away. This allows for acceptance of the moment as it is, fostering a sense of calm in both body and mind, which nurtures a lasting relationship with your body.

Making Peace with This Moment

Body equanimity begins with accepting the present moment as it is, without judgment. As you learn to comfort and soothe uncomfortable sensations, emotions, and thoughts as they arise, your body and mind join together in letting go, revealing the peace you have been waiting to feel.

I don't know what you and your body need to let go of or make peace with right now. It might be years of body hatred or harm, internal dysregulation from feeling unsafe, or the impact of body oppression and stigma. It might be a current health situation or your body's physical abilities or the lack thereof. You might be struggling at this moment with how your body is aging, looking, or moving, or with how it can no longer move. You might be struggling with regrets from the past that resurface or with feeling another wave of grief.

Every moment is different. Sometimes you'll feel unburdened and think, "This is it! I'm done feeling this way!" Then regret or grief might return. There are moments of compassion, appreciation, and gratitude for your body—until it gets sick, requires extra care, or disappointment or betrayal surfaces again. This cycle is to be expected as you move toward living embodied, which is why letting go and finding body equanimity are so important.

Finding Steadiness in the Middle Ground

In Buddhist teachings equanimity is a balanced state of mind and body marked by an internal sense of steadiness. Body equanimity is about learning to be okay with how things are for your body in the moment, finding a balance where the experience is neither great nor a struggle. When you acknowledge and allow a challenging moment to simply exist, it transforms into something manageable. This middle ground is characteristic of equanimity. Each time you meet a moment this way, it feels like a release inside and brings you back to your center.

Body equanimity isn't about achieving a resolution or reaching an endpoint. It's not a one-time event, no matter what you're trying to release. Instead, it's a continual process of intention, release, and acceptance nurtured through forgiveness. Forgiving each intense or uncomfortable sensation, emotion, or thought is what shifts the moment from struggle to letting it be. My study participants called this shift the "okay moment."

This Moment Is Okay

Call to mind your last challenging moment with your body when you found yourself to be in old, familiar patterns of sensations, emotions, and thoughts over something you thought you were done with. When you have a moment in mind, answer the following questions:

1. What instigated the challenging moment?

2. What familiar sensations, emotions, and thoughts came up?

3. As you reflect, notice if any sensations, emotions, or thoughts are here with you now.

4. Place one hand on your heart and the other hand on your belly below your navel. Connect with your center by gently rocking or swaying side to side or front to back. Say out loud or to yourself:

I hoped these moments wouldn't return, but they still do.
May I return to my center, my internal equanimity.

These moments will come again and again, whether I want them to or not.
May I return to my center, my internal equanimity.

I am allowed to not feel okay in these moments.
May I return to my center, my internal equanimity.

It's okay not to feel okay sometimes. All living things sometimes don't feel okay.
May I return to my center, my internal equanimity.

I don't have to fight or change this moment.
May I return to my center, my internal equanimity.

This moment is okay. It's neither great nor does it have
to be. It just is.
May I return to my center, my internal equanimity.

This moment may feel like the past, but it's different
from the past.
May I return to my center, my internal equanimity.

This moment can be okay.

It's not easy to let a moment be without trying to change it, especially when you're scared or off-center. But each time you nurture equanimity, you cultivate body forgiveness.

Body Equanimity Creates Space for Choice

When a difficult body moment softens into being okay, you'll notice your mind softens too. Creating space around intense experiences gives you the chance to reevaluate the moment and see it with more clarity. This is your body returning to center—your place of grounding. From here, you can reason, make different choices, and see new possibilities. What once felt impossible can become doable. Where your thoughts were headed down to dysfunction junction, filled with what's impossible, now there are multiple open roads.

Through equanimity, you can accept that messages from your body—whether your mind labels them "good" or "bad," "pleasant" or "unpleasant"—are simply forms of embodied information. Meg, a study participant, described it this way: "I had to recognize the physical manifestations of the messages in my body. I feel my mind connects with the physical manifestations and understands them better now. I no longer judge them as an interference with life. They are life!"

Approaching these signals with equanimity allows you to interpret them in a new way. Recently I had heart palpitations, which usually means my thyroid medication needs adjusting. But as I age, a racing heart scares me. My mind started to spiral: "Oh no, do I have a heart condition? Not another thing!" I softened and connected with my body through equanimity, reminding myself, "I don't have to like or dislike this moment. This moment of fear can be okay." That brought me back to center. My mind opened up to possibilities: "I'll call my endocrinologist tomorrow. Maybe I just need to adjust my medication." By addressing one message at a time, you can work toward understanding what your body needs and maybe even contribute to its healing.

Holding the Intention to Rebuild Trust

Body equanimity and rebuilding body safety go hand in hand. When sensations, thoughts, or emotions are met with equanimity, your nervous system stays regulated and your thoughts stay clear and focused on the moment, not hijacked by the past or the future. Only when you let go of what you are holding on to can you rebuild trust and create the healing needed for a new relationship with your body.

Rebuilding safety starts with intentional focus, constantly reminding yourself of the relationship you want with your body. The question "What do I aspire to build?" helps you reconnect to your body and build a more secure relationship with it every time you face intense sensations, emotions, or thoughts. Intentional focus allows you to pause, reassess, and refocus on what matters most—a deeper, more embodied connection. Instead of engaging with painful memories that led to body hatred, shame, and blame, Joyse, a study participant, shared: "I had to relax into the moment and remind myself that maybe this is not in line with my highest good, and I let go of all the coulds, woulds, shoulds, and if onlys. . . . this leaves me more expansive and opens up what's possible."

By focusing on the relationship you aspire to, you can reevaluate and gain a new understanding of challenging experiences. Joyse's insight came from recognizing that her current moment didn't align with her aspiration. She forgave the moment, which brought softness, release, and space around her memories and emotions. This equanimity let her realign with what mattered: her nervous system resetting, her mind calming, and her body returning to center. It's not your fault that memories and ideas resurface. Through equanimity and forgiveness, you can allow these moments, soften into being okay, and move forward.

How Body Equanimity Supports Your Relationship with Food

In chapter 2 you looked at your body's relationship with food, which was once a neutral source of nourishment. Over time this relationship may have shifted. What was once nourishing can now create fear, confusion, and dysregulation. Body equanimity helps you imagine a new way to relate to food—a steady, balanced state where all foods are acceptable and you understand that some foods provide more ease and balance while others may not. Equanimity lets both ideas coexist.

You're constantly receiving external messages about food, but you can choose to trust your body's signals over those external messages. A more harmonious relationship with food begins with attuning to your body's interoceptive signals. The next time you feel conflicted about food, pause and reflect: Is this coming from your mind or your body?

Most food fears—unless they're about allergies or sensitivities—are rooted in the mind and influenced by diet culture. Notice how your body responds to foods you see as threatening. What does your body have to say about these foods? For example, with celiac disease, when I eat gluten my body sends clear signals of discomfort, including pain, bloating, and malaise. But as a teen I avoided French fries because the diet culture said fried foods were bad. My friends enjoyed sharing the French fries, but I chose cottage cheese and fruit. My mind's fear, not my body, kept me from enjoying moments of connection and joy with friends at the late-night diner. Once I started eating fries again (as long as they were gluten-free), my body responded with ease and equanimity.

EMBODIED PRACTICE

Allowing Your Body to Decide

Try this at meals to develop a more equanimous relationship with food:

1. At your next meal, pause and notice your food choices. What drew you to these foods—your body or your mind? Did fear or internalized messages influence you? What might your body wish for instead? Notice what's happening inside as you ask these questions.

2. Place one hand on your heart and the other below your navel. Connect with your center by gently rocking or swaying, side to side or front to back, and say:
   I can soften and allow my body to make new choices.

   My body can choose based on internal ease and connection over fear.

   My body gets to choose, not just my mind.

Interoceptive listening helps you discern what food your body truly desires based on inner truth rather than fear, giving you and your body the agency you've been waiting for.

Releasing the Moment Allows You to Stay in the Moment

An internal shift happens when you face uncomfortable sensations, emotions, and thoughts with equanimity. Pausing and connecting with your body during discomfort fosters safety and presence, encouraging exploration over avoidance. The study participant Jeanne-Marie said, "To feel what I need from the inside, I have to stop, drop in, and roll around in there for a while!"

Your body may signal release through softening, tears, relaxed muscles, openness, lightness, reduced fear, or physical movements like shaking, all while your mind quiets. Here's what other study participants shared about their experience with equanimity:

"There is a softening. Things shift but I don't have to make them shift."—MAGGIE

"The tightness releases. Allowing the moment to be okay keeps the compassionate connection between me and my body. It keeps the 'we' [tears flow]."—SARA

"Stillness, relaxed and supported."—LISA

"Expansive and opening up."—JOYSE

"Becoming lighter."—EVE

"Letting go of the vigilance, release."—AMELIA

"I shake, move, swim. It's a constant. I can't think about it. It's not from the mind. It's happening all the time. Something inside moves and shifts."—SOPHIA

"A relaxation in my body. Not so tightly held."—MEG

"When the release is in my fingers and toes I don't have to do the analysis. My body helps facilitate the letting go."—PEARL

EMBODIED PRACTICE

Somatically Releasing Tough Moments

Try the following release practices and see which calls to you most. Use any of them the next time you're in a challenging moment:

1. Lie on your back with your legs long and about three feet apart. Windshield wiper your feet back and forth several times. Start slow, quicken the pace, then slow down again. Pause and notice the shifting sensation in your legs and body.

2. Lying down or sitting, open and close your hands quickly for a count of five. Pause and open your fingers wide for five seconds. Repeat. Shake out your hands and rest them, palms open, noticing the shifting sensation in your hands and body.

3. Stand with your feet three feet apart. Open your arms out to the side, breathe in, exhale, and cross your arms over your chest, placing your hands on the opposite shoulders, giving yourself a hug. Repeat with the other arm on top. End with arms wide open and notice the shifting sensations.

4. Sit on the ground or in a chair and hug your knees to your chest. Slowly rock back and forth, side to side, and front to

back. Let your head soften toward your knees. Slow
down and notice the shifting sensations in your head,
neck, and body.

The Power of Sustaining Attention

Embracing body equanimity and allowing the moment to be as it is
helps you reconnect with your body's internal experience and regain
a sense of safety and agency after stressful moments. In chapter 4
you learned that your body produces a stress response when faced
with challenges. Increasing interoceptive awareness allows you to
link your sensations, emotions, and thoughts, leading to insights
that interrupt the stress cycle and bring you back to your center.
Dr. Price calls this practice of cultivating awareness "sustaining
attention."[2]

Staying with Your Body During Challenging Times

This practice is available as an audio recording at www.shambhala
.com/body-forgiveness-practices.

PART ONE

Recall a recent challenging moment. Select a moment that rates no
higher than a five on a scale of one to ten for trauma sensitivity. (This
practice can be revisited with more challenging situations as you
develop the capacity to sustain focus.) Consider how this moment
may have left you feeling unsafe or overwhelmed by sensory cues,
thoughts, or emotional responses.

1. Sit comfortably and close your eyes or keep a soft, relaxed gaze.

2. Reach your arms overhead and inhale. Exhale and let your arms release alongside your body. Repeat this several times.

3. Recall the challenging moment. Notice how it lands in your body. What sensory cues do you notice? Does your heart rate change? Is there tension? Where do you notice it?

4. Pause and identify the area that needs your attention most. Place a hand there or use a pillow or bolster if needed.

5. Take a breath and say, *I see you, feel you, and sense you. I am here.*

6. Soften your thoughts, asking your mind for permission to be right here with this sensation. What's it like inside this space?

7. Be curious. What happens when you "stop, drop in, and roll around" in this space? What's happening inside?

8. If an emotion is present within, can you meet it with equanimity, allowing it to be with you?

9. Can you rest here with the emotion and sensation, attending to what you observe and feel? No need to rush. If your attention wanders, shift or move slightly, then refocus. Lean in to listen to your body.

10. If a part of you feels unsure or unsafe, ask permission to rest here for a while, assuring the part that feels unsafe that this isn't forever.

11. Notice if bringing compassion and equanimity into the experience helps you stay grounded. Any sense of softening or release is a sign of returning to center.

12. Observe any changes within this space. Have sensations within and around it shifted in any way?

13. Are you forming awareness or discovery by staying with your body's sensations and emotions? If so, allow that to develop as you rest within here. There's no need to rush away. Your body needs you to stay here.

14. Once you feel calm and connected, gently release your touch, knowing you can return anytime.

PART TWO

After the practice, journal on these questions:

- What was the challenging situation?

- Where did you notice it in your body?

- What sensations stood out the most?

- How did you quiet your mind to stay with your body?

- Were you able to sustain your focus? What did you notice? Any emotions, memories, or shifts?

- Did you make any connections between your sensory, emotional, mental, and spiritual bodies?

- How might you use these connections to further your relationship with your body?

Equanimity enables you to access and maintain sustained focus, and sustained focus fosters greater equanimity, creating a cycle of ease. As you grow in awareness and self-understanding, your body will no longer feel foreign, and sensations won't evoke the same fears.

Accepting That Your Body Will Change

One of the biggest challenges of being embodied is facing the inevitability of body change. Our bodies are impermanent, just like everything else. We're born, we live, we age, and eventually we die. For some, accepting this is difficult. Others, perhaps through illness or brushes with death, may have come to terms with it. Every day as embodied beings we face impermanence.

Impermanence (Pali: *anicca*) is a core Buddhist teaching. Attachment to the belief that you can control your body to keep it the same causes suffering. By accepting your body's ever-changing nature, you can let go of this attachment and end suffering. But even if you understand this intellectually, it's still hard to embrace, especially as a woman in a culture that threatens invisibility and disregard when your body changes to no longer be the ideal size, shape, age, ability, and health.

Your body changing isn't your body's fault, it's simply its nature. But change is scary and uncertain, and your mind doesn't like that. It wants to figure out and make sense of what's happening. Equanimity, fueled by compassion and forgiveness, reminds you it's okay not to like the changes your body is undergoing. Your body may not appreciate them either! Change is hard for both body and mind. When the two-time Women's National Basketball Association's Most Valuable Player Elena Delle Donne retired, she said, "My body seemed to make this decision before my mind accepted it."[3] Her words imply that her interoceptive signals helped her recognize this body truth before her mind accepted it, which illustrates how challenging it can be to accept the inevitable changes our bodies undergo.

Body Change Is an Opportunity to Grieve

Most body changes are another moment of grief and require grieving. I wish I could say you will reach a point where change is no longer scary or throws you off-center, but that wouldn't be true.

We suffer this way because we're human beings in ever-changing bodies.

Sometimes you can predict changes—for example, during pregnancy. Most of the time, however, changes occur unexpectedly, as when an illness or injury suddenly happens. While writing this chapter, I was diagnosed with another autoimmune illness. When I began the book I mostly felt healthy. Midway through my condition shifted. I noticed new signals from my body. At first I felt gripping sensations, a tight stomach, and racing thoughts. Questions flooded my mind: "Did I do something to bring this on? Could I have done something differently? What does this mean for my future?" These questions only threw me off-center, creating fear and further internal dysregulation, and pulling me away from my body's present experience. By practicing equanimity and focusing on my body's sensations, I realized my body was feeling better that day even if my mind wasn't.

This was another moment of grief. I forgave myself for feeling scared and forgave my body for developing another illness. I reminded myself that my body didn't ask for this either. We're in this together. Once I acknowledged my body's change with compassion and forgiveness, my mind softened and grief moved into grieving.

You Can Either Accept or Resist Your Body's Evolution

From birth, your body changes significantly—why wouldn't it? It's no different than any living organism. Your body evolves through every experience, just as every living thing does. Depending on your age, this evolution may represent a significant part of your life and be filled with many transformations.

Ask yourself: *How have I met these transformations? Have I allowed or resisted my body's changes?* Allowing your body to change means respecting its impermanent nature. Unfortunately, women are often taught to resist and fight against natural changes, to try to control them. One question I ask clients with disordered eating is if they've ever discovered their body's natural weight and size. Most women have no idea, because disembodiment and attempts to change the body have gone on so long.

Resisting your body's evolution often leads to body manipulation—changing your appearance, size, shape, or functioning through diet, exercise, surgery, or anti-aging products. Years ago I read Sogyal Rinpoche's *The Tibetan Book of Living and Dying*, which introduced me to body impermanence. In Tibetan the word for "body" is *lu*, meaning something you leave behind, like baggage. He reminds us that the body is impermanent, and we're just travelers taking "temporary refuge in this life and in this body." He likens our obsession with improving our bodies to "redecorating a hotel room every time we check in."[4]

Since recovering from an eating disorder and practicing and living embodiment for more than thirty-five years, I no longer manipulate my body through exercise or diet. But I still "redecorate" daily—I wear makeup, dye my hair, try to minimize wrinkles, and look for vitamins to help me live longer. I accept this redecorating project with compassion and joy, knowing this body is temporary and not my true home. What brings peace is embracing my body's internal messages, accepting its constant changes, and embracing its impermanent nature.

As you age it's also natural to wonder how your relationship with your body might have been different if you'd learned to listen to it earlier or been taught to accept its changes as natural. The next reflection gives you a chance to understand your body's transformation and offer forgiveness to yourself for not knowing how to listen sooner.

My Body's Transformation

Reflect on your body's evolution and how it's shifted, changed, and tried to communicate with you over the years.

CHILDHOOD: This is a time of accelerated body change. You went from being entirely dependent to walking, talking, and eating on your own. How did your body shift and change during these years of rapid growth? How much was natural progression and how much was the result of external manipulation and forced change (by yourself or others)? What messages did your body try to communicate?

ADOLESCENCE: This is another significant period in our lives, marked by a dramatic shift in hormones and maturation that often produces significant body changes. In what ways did your body shift and change? How much was natural progression and how much was the result of external manipulation and forced change? What messages did your body try to communicate?

YOUNG ADULTHOOD: This time is often marked by many external changes in our lives. Relationships may be forming or ending. Life transitions that produce changing stress levels, such as college and work, come into play. In what ways did your body shift and change? How much was natural progression and how much was the result of external manipulation and forced change? What messages did your body try to communicate?

ADULTHOOD: This period tends to bring on many more stressors that may leave us feeling off-center. Hormones may be shifting again and you may be expending energy caring and attending for others. In what ways did your body shift and change? How much was natural progression and how much was the result of external manipulation and forced change? What messages did your body try to communicate?

MIDDLE ADULTHOOD: Our bodies begin to show signs of aging and may start sending signals of internal changes in organ functioning and hormone levels. In what ways did your body shift and change? How much was natural progression and how much was the result of external manipulation and forced change? What messages did your body try to communicate?

LATER ADULTHOOD: Like childhood and adolescence, this is also a time of rapid body change. As our bodies continue to age, we may encounter challenges that we are not accustomed to. Our bodies may have additional needs that require attention and care. In what ways did your body shift and change? How much was natural progression and how much was the result of external manipulation and forced change? What messages did your body try to communicate?

Place a hand on your heart. Sway or rock your body. Let grief turn into grieving and allow equanimity and compassion to emerge. Say to yourself, *I'm not sure if I listened or have given you everything you needed at each stage of life. If I could have done it differently, I would have.*

Accepting Your Body's Changes Requires a Different Response

Accepting change and uncertainty in your body requires a radically different approach. To accept your body as it is, you must let it be as it is. Acceptance, like forgiveness, can't come from the mind—it must come from the heart. That means letting go and grieving what your body once was and what you hoped it would be and instead focusing on how it is right now. Gail, a study participant, said, "I no longer resist my body's messages and changes; I just let them move and flow and ask, 'Oh, what are you teaching me now?' I've learned that it's not just about my body's changes, but about my response to my body's changes!"

As your body changes, it tries to communicate through sensory messages. Sometimes you listen, especially when the messages are loud, like pain. Sometimes you push through and ignore them. Recognizing that you've been bypassing body messages for so long can lead to grief and regret. It's essential to meet this with self-compassion. Remind yourself, *Of course I didn't listen. I didn't know how, and external messages encouraged me not to!* Our culture encourages moving past, pushing through, and bypassing negative sensory information at all costs.

Accepting your body's impermanence means developing a new response to these sensory messages. For example, you can forgive yourself for repeatedly wishing your body were different and allowing these feelings and thoughts to resurface even when you believe you have moved past them. You can forgive yourself for wanting your body to perform differently and for wanting it to feel better. You can also forgive your body for changing. Your body never meant to cause you any harm by changing. It's always been trying to evolve, just like all living things.

Your Body's Evolution

1. Close your eyes or soften your gaze.

2. Take a few release breaths. Place a hand on your heart and the other on your navel—your midpoint, your center.

3. Focus inside the space between your hands, navel to heart and heart to navel.

4. Soften and let these words settle into this space:
    My body is a mystery.
    It evolves and changes as all living things do.
    May I soften and allow my body to evolve and change.
    May I soften and allow my body to evolve and change just as all living things are allowed to.

This chapter helps you appreciate and respect your body's mysteries and changes, which fosters peace. Pause and reflect on the changes you are noticing. Are you feeling more at peace within your body? Perhaps a new softening and acceptance toward your body is developing, as well as a more compassionate understanding that, like all living beings, your body will change over time. Cultivating body equanimity supports you through these transitions, letting you gently let go, forgive, grieve, and reconnect with a body that's been waiting for you your whole life.

I'm okay with what's next. My work for today is to just figure myself out for today.

—**MARTHA, STUDY PARTICIPANT**

10

EMBRACING EMBODIMENT

Living an Embodied Life

> I am learning how not to think but to pray and use my body
> to access the sacred—to locate the sacred of my own body.[1]
> —LEKEY LEIDECKER

THE TENTH AND FINAL STAGE of body forgiveness is about embracing what it truly means to be embodied and to live an embodied life. Like forgiveness, living in an embodied way doesn't come from your mind, it comes from intentionally committing to a relationship with your body from the heart—acknowledging and responding to your body in each moment, all while being held in compassion and forgiveness.

Experiencing Embodiment from Within

Throughout this book, you've learned what it takes to develop a new relationship with your body—one that helps you understand yourself and identify what you and your body need at any given moment. This chapter explores how to remain committed to this relationship and truly embody what it means to live with your body from a subjective, not objective, view.

Living with your body as a subject means moving beyond seeing your body as an object. Instead, you witness your body through a profound connection that is both sensory and spiritual, recognizing you and your body as one, with no separation. As old thought patterns about your body's needs, wants, and desires diminish, they're replaced by respect, understanding, cooperation, and a newfound sense of oneness. You'll discover that between you and your body, there is something more profound than mere thoughts. As the study participant Sofie expressed, "It's when I bring my soul to connect with my body. It's when my body connects with my spirit." Another study participant, Jean-Marie, said, "I'm not separate. There's an energetic connection [always present] if I can open my heart to my body."

Their words echo the wisdom of Indigenous peoples, mystics, sages, and early philosophers who knew there is no separation between mind, body, and spirit. In many ways, embodiment is a homecoming—a return to the wholeness and interconnectedness of your body. Practicing the exercises in this book will give you a new, subjective, and relational perspective that will help you begin this journey.

The We Experience

The stages of body forgiveness help you move from seeing your body as separate—or even as an enemy—to recognizing it as an integral part of yourself. This final stage invites you to see your body in unity with you. I call this "the we experience." When you engage in the we experience, you acknowledge your commitment to your body. Like any committed relationship, this declaration becomes an anchor to lean on when tough moments arise. Instead of running away during challenges, you become aware of what pulls you away and how to return. You no longer feel troubled by distractions because you know these moments are normal and you'll come back into relationship with your body again. This relationship is grounded in the security and peace of knowing you and your body are committed to staying connected. Amelia, a study participant, described this as an unwavering relationship with a good-enough quality that leaves her feeling safe. Sarah called the we experience a welcoming home, expressing her desire to keep returning to that place.

Even with a strong commitment to the we experience, feeling connected to your body will still vary day to day. This is natural—external circumstances, changes in your body's needs, and your emotions and thoughts can all disrupt your sense of ease. You may lose this connection and need to rediscover it again and again, and that's perfectly okay. From now on, you can let go of the idea that this connection is perfect—because there's no such thing! Living embodied doesn't have to be a struggle; it's about trusting that this relationship is always growing and evolving, and that it will be imperfect. This process continues until your body and spirit transcend past death and into the next dimension.

There are no strict rules for living an embodied life. It's about feeling and sensing when you're truly present in the connection and recognizing what supports you during challenging times—just like any stable, secure relationship. The following reflection helps you explore this commitment.

EMBODIED REFLECTION

Where You Have Been and Where You Are Now

Pause here. Slow down in your body. Shift your seat side to side, or if you're standing, come to a steady stance. Take a deep breath in and release it with a big sigh, making an "ahhh" sound. Reflect on the changes you've felt unfold between you and your body so far.

- What shifts have you noticed most since the start of this book?

- How has your understanding of your body changed?

- How has your kindness and compassion toward your body shifted?

- How has your relationship with forgiving and allowing you and your body to grieve changed?

- How has your ability to remain present with your body changed? Are you finding you can attune to your body and what it needs?

- How has your relationship with letting go and allowing your body to sometimes not be okay changed?

- Are you noticing more within your body? How have you become more sensory aware and connected?

No matter where you are on this journey, you've progressed in your relationship with your body—even if you're just noticing little glimmers of awareness starting to blossom. Take a deep breath in and release it with a big sigh. You and your body have learned a lot and have done everything you could together up to this point. If you're willing and curious, take the next step in your commitment to each other—there's still more to explore and discover.

Staying Curious Helps You Stay Connected

Living embodied means actively addressing the habitual patterns of your mind that hinder deeper connection. Remember, your body exists only in the present moment, continuously experiencing life as it unfolds—like young children, who approach everything with wonder and a fresh perspective. Habitual thoughts often make us forget this essential truth.

You may have recognized thoughts that interfere with living fully in your body, like self-criticism or rumination. But it's also important to notice subtler thoughts that can disrupt your connection, especially when you're about to do something positive for your body—enjoy a favorite meal, shop for new clothes, or participate in a joyful activity. Sometimes old programmed thoughts flood in to stop you. This is when mindfulness and the balanced energy you learned about in chapter 5 can help you show up with full intention to be present in your body.

Adopting the perspective of "we are in this together" is especially helpful in these moments. Sometimes you need this perspective to be strong, like a loving but firm parent. Sarah, one of the study participants, shared that when she feels disconnected and on the verge of slipping back into old habits, she quickly asserts, "Nope, we are not doing this anymore! Things have changed and we are trying."

While writing this chapter I experienced a flare-up of my autoimmune disorder. I felt lightheaded and fatigued, to the point where I had to stop writing. I noticed disconnection starting, along with fearful thoughts: "What if I can't finish the manuscript? What if this gets worse?" As those thoughts spiraled, I acknowledged them and countered with a loving but firm reminder: "No, fearful thoughts won't help me now. I'm not going there. What does my body wish to tell me instead?" This loving firmness helped me drop beneath my mind back to curiosity about my body's experience.

What would it be like now to let your body guide you back to its messages?

Deepening Curiosity for Your Body's Messages

In my research on body forgiveness, one word stood out about living and returning to embodiment: *curiosity*. Disconnection and moments of feeling disconnected from your body are to be expected. What matters now is developing curiosity during those moments. Staying curious about your body helps you feel more connected and regain that connection when external forces, emotions, and thoughts disrupt it. Curiosity includes being interested in your habitual thoughts, bodily messages, and the expression and allowance of emotions.

Staying curious about the messages your body is communicating through interoception—your internal awareness—helps you stay connected through a felt sense rather than trying to think your way back. As the study participant Martha said, "It has to be a felt understanding to bring yourself back. It's a thing happening in the moment. You have to stay with what you notice to bring yourself back."

As you've learned, difficult moments are just that—difficult! They often lead to dysregulation and make you feel off-center. Habitual sensations in your body—pain, tension, a racing heart, and feeling stuck or collapsed—may return. These are crucial times to acknowledge and name your internal experience. You can focus and sustain your attention toward your body, as you learned in chapter 9, by taking a breath and saying, *I see you, feel you, and sense you. I am here.*

Soften your thoughts by asking your busy mind for permission to be right here with this sensation. What's it like inside during this challenging moment? Get curious about the sensations. What happens when you stop, drop in, and roll around inside your body's experience for a while? What do you notice in this moment of disconnection?

During my own moment of disconnection, I was aware of my thoughts and asked my fearful mind for permission to soften them so I could focus on the underlying messages. I noticed my lower back felt inflamed and achy—a familiar sensation. I named it "inflammation in my back." Even though I'd hoped it wouldn't return, it had. Self-compassion reminded me that my body doesn't like this discomfort either. I recommitted to my body, realizing it needed relief. I placed a pillow under my back, and the softness helped redirect my attention inward. I envisioned the fatigue in my back—hot, heavy, and red. By leaning into my body and listening instead of overthinking, I understood it was communicating a need for a break. My body felt sad about going through this again too.

What would it be like now to recognize, in each uncomfortable moment, that your body is sad about experiencing this again too?

What Is Your Body Communicating?

This reflection helps you notice and name your internal experience, allowing you to remain embodied and keep the lines of communication open with your body.

- Call to mind a recent moment of body disconnection.

- Soften your thoughts and invite your busy mind to be present with the sensations that arose during that moment and may be arising again now.

- What messages did you receive from your body? Was there a shift in your internal energy? Are there particular sensations that stood out and may stand out? Are any of these same sensations and changes in your internal energy happening again now?

- Can you allow yourself to be curious about these sensations without criticism? Remind yourself that you and your body are in this challenge together. Place one hand over your heart and the other beneath your navel to reconnect with your center. Repeat: *I know my body is trying to tell me something. I know my body may not like these recurring sensations either. Can I continue to listen?*

Staying Curious About Your Emotional Experiences

Difficult thoughts, sensations, and emotions often arise together during challenging moments with your body. These moments can bring up grief, fear, shame, embarrassment, frustration, anger, resentment, and hopelessness. It's understandable that when old challenges resurface, the same emotions will too. Acknowledging these emotions helps your body and mind not be caught off guard.

Remember, emotions and expressing emotions are natural to your body. These moments signify a longing to let emotions flow freely. The study participant Pearl expressed this perfectly when she said, "I have to ask: What is keeping me stuck? What is the holdup? I know that freedom and ease await on the other side." When emotions are allowed to move through, relief is often waiting.

As I lay on the ground, focusing on my sensory experience, I noticed that the more I paused and slowed down, giving comfort to my body through sustained attention and presence, the more emotions surfaced—eager to be acknowledged and felt so they could flow. My eyes filled with tears. I reminded myself that tears mean my body is trying to return to homeostasis and unblock the river of emotion. I let the tears flow, not needing to know exactly what I was feeling. Once the emotions released and I returned to my center, I could become curious about what was present. There were familiar feelings of fear, sadness, and grief, but I also noticed feelings of helplessness and vulnerability—new emotions that are likely a response to this new diagnosis and my aging body.

What would it be like now to allow emotions to be a fluid sensory experience within your body?

Emotions Are Meant to Be Fluid

This reflection creates space around challenging emotions by pausing, slowing down, embodying, and letting them flow freely, helping you reconnect with your body.

- Use the moment of body disconnection in the previous reflection.

- Notice the felt sense of emotions that arose and may arise again. Are they familiar or new?

- Begin to sway or rock your body, inviting it to meet the internal river of emotions that wants to move freely.

- Use the visual image of a river, as in chapter 4. Can these emotions find their way over, below, or around anything in their way?

- Can you approach these emotions with compassion and curiosity, without judgment?

- Place one hand over your heart and the other beneath your navel to reconnect with your center. Repeat: *But of course my body and I feel this again. Why wouldn't we? I can feel this and still come back. We can feel this together.*

You Are Allowed to Take a Body Break

As I age, I often joke, "My body is like a Rolls-Royce—it requires a lot of management, maintenance, and care!" The truth is, my body does need attention, and some days I get tired of the upkeep. On one recent day like this, even though my body signaled me to wake up and stretch, I chose to stay in bed past my alarm. Maybe I'll get to my practice later, maybe I won't. My body and I may be uncomfortable today, but we're still okay. Just like in any committed relationship, time apart doesn't threaten the relationship.

When you need a break, check in—maybe what you really need is to let the river of emotion flow. I've found that when I need a break, I need to let grief move into grieving again and again.

As you move forward, remember there will be days when you don't want to attend to your body's needs, and that's perfectly okay. Keep in mind the wisdom of the study participant Sophia: "The only rule is NO rule!" When you've had enough of your body's demands, consciously step back from it and know your body will forgive you. Its nature is compassionate and forgiving.

Setting Boundaries Can Help Your Emotions Flow

Boundaries are your and your body's clear, porous safety net, protecting what you both need. They help strengthen your relationship and commitment to your body by communicating, "We've got this!"

A porous boundary means you don't have to block anything out entirely. Instead, you create a circle of space that neither shuts out nor lets in too much. When a boundary is set with equanimity, it feels clear and intentional, not reactive. Now is the time to pay attention to what boundaries your body needs to feel safe—within your environment, with others, and with yourself. You might visualize a boundary as a net that surrounds you, allowing emotions to flow and your needs to be expressed freely.

WITHIN YOU: A boundary within your body needs both a visual aid and an internal felt sense. Pause and gently rock or sway. Place one hand on your heart and the other on your abdomen below your navel. Focus on your center and visualize the part of you, no matter how small, that cannot be taken away, influenced, or manipulated.

Let an image or color emerge from this felt sense. Name this space: "Nothing can take this from within me." Many years ago, during yoga therapy training, I discovered my internal visual aid—an image of a stake in the ground supporting my back body. I rely on this image whenever I need to feel safe and protected.

AROUND YOU: Consider how your environment supports your commitment to your body. Do you have a time or space at home or elsewhere that allows you to feel at ease? For example, when you are in the shower, driving in your car, or sitting in a park. Say out loud, "This is our space." You may even decide to give it a name. By naming and claiming it, you allow your mind, body, and spirit to align. It is in these defined moments that you can access a sense of something greater than yourself to protect you and your body. For me, I feel at ease in a small area in my bedroom dedicated to my meditation and yoga practice. Even though it's a shared space, when I sit on my cushion or roll out my mat, it feels like it belongs to me and my body.

WITH OTHERS: Relational boundaries can be challenging because they require you to recognize when you're prioritizing someone else's needs over your own and those of your body. Boundary-setting within relationships is essential for ongoing embodiment. In chapter 6 you were encouraged to use this phrase during difficult relational moments: *May I give this to myself so that I may give to another.* It's essential to remind yourself that it's okay to prioritize your own needs first; doing so enables you to support others adequately. By setting boundaries and prioritizing your needs, you strengthen your commitment and relationship with your body.

As a helping professional for thirty-five years, I've learned to prior-itize my own needs and my body's needs. As my body's needs have changed, so have my office hours. I used to sit for long stretches to see multiple clients a day, but now my body can't tolerate that and my mind feels fatigued. I've learned to set boundaries with others to accommodate my changing body.

Staying Curious About What Brings You Back

The most important and compassionate thing to remember for your journey to embodiment is that disconnection will happen. We all experience moments of disconnection. What matters most is recognizing what brings you back. The key is discovering what helps you reconnect once you recognize you've become disconnected.

My study participants found that various activities helped them reconnect, including being in nature, feeling their breath during yoga, saying a prayer, pausing to ground themselves, slowing down, engaging their senses, meditating, or immersing themselves in water. They valued quiet, restful moments as well as times of strength and active engagement with their bodies when they acknowledged and responded to sensations instead of bypassing them. This is a good time to pause and reflect on what helps you reconnect. Make a list of what you've noticed.

For me, when I feel disconnected I discover where tension is held in my body and meet it by supporting my body through gentle movement, restorative yoga poses, and mindful breathing. Lying down with a yoga bolster under my lower back provides a sense of sturdiness, grounding, and steadiness that I was missing.

What would it be like now to explore and experience what brings you back to grounding and steadiness within?

Connecting from Head to Toe

This practice encourages slow, steady, grounded movement to reconnect with your body. If meditation, prayer, or a mantra has helped you before, consider adding it.

1. Stand with your feet about three feet apart, or do this practice leaning against a wall or sitting if standing isn't accessible.

2. Take a few release breaths, in through your nose and out through your mouth.

3. Interlace your fingers and place your hands behind your head, cradling the back of your head. Gently press your hands into your head as you lean your head back, creating a countermovement. Gently rock your head. Stay here for a few breaths.

4. Release your hands and arms, shaking them out alongside your body.

5. Open your arms wide and cross arms to opposite sides of your body, like a big hug. Repeat several times.

6. Stomp one foot at a time into the ground, at any speed you choose.

7. Take a release breath. Stand still and notice the free-flowing energy in your body.

8. Repeat: *I am connected from head to toe. There is something safe and bigger than me inside my body. I am not alone. My body is my home.*

Discovering an Embodied Relationship with Food

Throughout this book you've been exploring a new relationship with your body's first nurturer: food. Now is the time to become even more curious about this relationship. What changes are you noticing? Are you letting your body determine what it wants to eat and when? This is crucial for living an embodied life.

What would it be like to let your food choices be guided by your body's internal, interoceptive knowledge? After each meal or food choice, pause, lean into your body, and listen to its messages. In chapter 3 you imagined what it could be like if food were once again comforting, soothing, safe, and protective. How does it feel now?

What Is Your Relationship with Food Now?

- Reflect on these questions each time you make a food choice. That may seem like a lot of reflecting, and I know this may still be hard. Compassionately remember that returning to an embodied relationship with food takes time. However, each time you check in with your body before, during, and after a meal, you are building the we experience.

- Who decides what you and your body eat now? Someone or something outside, or are decisions made from within? Do we get to decide together?

- As you lean in and listen, what sensory messages let you know this food choice left you both feeling connected?

- Did the choices bring comfort to your body and mind? What sensory messages let you know this?

- After these choices, do we feel connected? If not, how might we do this differently next time?

Living with Embodied Acceptance

Embodied acceptance is crucial for reconnecting with your body. It's more than accepting your body's appearance; it means embracing your body's changes with curiosity and interest while attuning and responding to its needs.

Here is what some of the study participants said about acceptance. Gail shared, "I've learned to accept changes just like I would with anything that changes rapidly, like a puppy. It's both challenging and interesting at the same time!" Sophia said, "It has to be intuitive on a day-to-day basis, fluid and responsive." Rebecca added, "My body is going through its changes whether I want it to or not. I accept them because I don't want to miss out on anything."

Meg defined embodied acceptance as the ability to "experience everything from your body without avoiding it any longer." Jean-Marie said, "I don't have to like what's happening right now but acknowledging that this is happening is a form of acceptance!"

EMBODIED PRACTICE

Accepting Your Body in a New Way

This meditation helps you accept the changes, challenges, and needs that your body may be experiencing right now. You may do this practice sitting or lying down.

Place one hand on your heart and the other on your abdomen below your navel to connect with your center. Say the following phrases to your body:

I know you have changed and will continue to change. I acknowledge your changes.

I know you have changed and will continue to change. I am softening and surrendering to your changes.

I know you have changed and will continue to change. I will stay curious and interested in what you now need from me.

I will look after you. We are in this together now.

Reconnecting Through Embodied Movement

I have been a yoga teacher for nearly twenty years and a yoga therapist for over a decade. Today, I refer to myself as an embodiment teacher. This reflects my passion for helping people reconnect with their embodied experience through movement. Embodied movement means leaning into your body and listening to its messages to discern what movements it wants to make. There's no prescribed plan—it's just you and your body.

At first this may feel strange. You might wonder, "What should I do? How do I start?" We're conditioned to control our movement with our minds and to dutifully follow the instructions of others. This leads us to miss opportunities for exploration and imagination. Rather than look for external direction, begin by paying attention to your body's nature and instincts.

In Buddhist teachings and in Ayurvedic and Chinese medicine, we're encouraged to see our bodies as made of the same elements as nature: earth, air, fire, and water. These elements can be observed in nature and felt within us. We're born from this world, and when we die our bodies will return to it.

Connecting with nature's elements within your body is a great way to explore embodied movement. The following reflection and practice help you identify which element you're most drawn to.

Embodying Nature Within

We embody the earth element as density, hardness, solidity, and firmness. Can you feel it in the density of your muscles, the layers and thickness of your skin, and the strength, solidity, and hardness of your bones? Notice the firmness of your vertebral column and the bones of your feet as they touch the ground. Where do you feel the earth element most strongly in your body? What's the center of your earth? What nourishes your body, mind, and spirit?

We embody the wind or air element as movement and change. Can you feel it in the change of temperature on your skin, in the movement of your breath and air within your body? Notice the flow of sensations, emotions, and thoughts. Where do you feel the wind or air element most strongly in your body? What helps you feel transparent, light, and free, untroubled in body and mind?

We embody the fire element in the fluctuation of temperature as we move between hot and cold, and as energy as we shift between overdrive, underdrive, and centered. Can you feel it in the acids of your stomach, in the activity of your digestive system, in the warmth of your lungs, or the heat of sexual impulses, along with your inner strength and boundaries? Where do you feel the fire element most strongly in your body? What ignites your feeling of aliveness and brings you vitality? What helps you to discern what you need and want most?

We embody the water element through the liquidity and cohesion present in our bodies. Our bodies are approximately 65 percent water. It's in your saliva, blood, mucus, and lymph. It lubricates the synovial fluid in your joints and keeps your fascia and connective tissues supple and elastic. Where do you feel the water element most strongly in your body? What helps you remain fluid in body, mind, and heart? What brings balance, virtue, and wisdom to your life and within your mind, body, and spirit?

Do you feel drawn to a particular element after reading its descriptions? Many of us are clear about which elements we prefer and which we do not. The following practice will help you discover each element through movement. Pay attention to the movements you are naturally attracted to. This may shift and change from day to day or throughout the seasons, depending on what your body needs most.

Moving Through the Elements

This practice is available as an audio recording at www.shambhala .com/body-forgiveness-practices. It begins lying down and eventually invites you to stand. As always, listen to what your body desires and modify the practice according to your body's needs.

1. Lie down on the ground or in your bed. Feel the support beneath you. Let your bones be heavy. Sense the earth element within you.

2. Imagine your breath moving down inside your bones—air moving within.

3. Move your arms and legs fluidly—circling, twisting, hugging, lifting in the way a baby might move its limbs. Let the water element come alive.

4. Let this movement grow larger to include your torso and spine. Notice temperature shifts as the fire element comes alive within your body.

5. Roll to the side and shift onto hands and knees, pressing into the ground, rocking and swaying, eventually standing up with feet firmly planted on the ground.

6. Let movement be spontaneous, inspired by earth, air, fire, and water elements. Your body guides you, reminding you: "We are here together, connected to all."

7. Sense each element alive within you: earth's firmness, air's lightness, fire's vitality, water's liquidity.

8. Which element calls to you the most? Can you let your body become this now? How does it want to move?

Notice images and memories that come alive as you and your body return to its embodied nature made up of the earth, wind, fire, and water.

Practice often until you notice which element you're drawn to the most and how it comes alive in your body. Let this guide your movement choices and be curious about how the elements you're drawn to can support other areas in your life, such as self-inquiry, food choices, or movement choices. For example, I'm most drawn to the elements of earth and water. With this awareness, I make sure my meals include the grounding energy of carbohydrates and grains as well as the water element found in fruits, vegetables, and dairy. I practice gentle yoga for joint and mind fluidity, sturdy yogic balance poses that allow me to feel the strength of my bones, and deep stretches for opening my connective tissue. I love walking by water, focusing on the rhythm of my feet as I take in the movement of the water around me. And I lift weights—my bones enjoying the grounding strength this produces, and my mind appreciating the fluidity of the repetition. I have learned that the balance of these elements within my body leaves me feeling more balanced in my life.

Embodied Movement Is Protective

The more you engage in embodied movement, the more you'll be guided by what feels natural to your body and its internal sensations rather than just your mind's ideas, which may still be influenced by diet culture and body image. As you move through any exercise or activity, ask: *What does this feel like inside?* and *What is my body telling me about this movement?* You might even declare, "I promise to engage only in movements that bring us vitality, strength, and groundedness."

Embodied movement helps you reconnect with your body as it changes, letting you adjust by being aware of your body's signals. Sometimes this means grieving what was. Practicing body equanimity lets you face these moments with compassion and acceptance. You can tell yourself, *This is okay*, so you can move forward and give your body what it needs.

After years of practicing headstands using a yogic headstand bench, my body messaged me through neck and shoulder pain that it was no longer right for me. I hesitated to sell the bench for a year, grieving the body I once had. During this time I let my emotions flow, practiced body equanimity, and embraced impermanence: "This is okay. My body is allowed to change. All living things change."

Returning Home

> I'm stunned that my body is still here. I'm awed by that. My body is not something other than me. What's saving my life right now and healing my life is the awareness and experience of the integral body and mind: the unity, inseparability, and integration of what we call body, mind, and spirit.
>
> —MAGGIE, STUDY PARTICIPANT

Take a deep breath and release it with an "ahhh." You've come a long way on your journey back to your body. Pause and notice even a glimmer of hope, pride, awe, or gratitude. No matter where you are on the path, you and your body are working together to create something new. You're both finding a new home together.

Moving Forward

Reflect on what you've learned and how you can best support yourself and your body moving forward. Journal or make an audio recording about the practices that have helped you most. Select a few that resonate now, as these will help you return to your center and reconnect with your body.

- Have you realized that you've always been searching for a way back home to your body, where you both feel safe, protected, and secure? What helps your body feel safe now?

- Have you come to understand that your body has its own spiritual path and journey, and that you may not be able to control its entire course? What supports you in accepting your body's unique journey?

- Have you grown to accept, from your heart, that some aspects of your body may change while others stay the same? What helps you embrace your body's changes?

- Have you recognized that the path ahead requires ongoing grieving, forgiving, and equanimity? What signals let you know that you need to grieve, forgive, or practice equanimity? What practices support you most?

- Can you accept that you may not heal all the wounds between you and your body, but that self-compassion can help prevent them from becoming worse? Place both hands to your heart and use the supportive mantra, *How can I not make this moment worse?* How does self-compassion support you?

Your body is—and has always been—a whole, living, feeling, sensing, and deeply interconnected spiritual entity. The separation that developed was just a misunderstanding. There is no "you" that exists separately from your body, and no body that exists apart from you.

Remembering You Are Not Alone

Even if it sometimes feels like it, you're not alone on this path. Embodiment and moments of living embodied remind us that we are interconnected and interdependent. From birth to death, we rely on others. Your body is no different; it needed care before your birth and will continue to need care throughout your life until it leaves this realm. The more connected you become with your body, the easier it is to remember your interconnectedness and your need to belong.

While contemporary culture may promote disembodiment and disconnection, you don't have to follow this trend. Many women, like you, are embracing the radical, countercultural movement toward somatic healing, embodiment, anti-diet practices, health at every size, body acceptance, body liberation, and protection for all bodies. You're not alone. But simply knowing this isn't enough; you need to seek out supportive messages and community. My study participants emphasized the importance of community and connection as the remedy for feeling alone. As Gail said, "A shared community helps me feel accepted."

Be mindful of what you absorb through TV, movies, music, and especially social media. Take time to clean up your feed. Unfollow accounts that make you feel alone or disconnected. Listen to what your body is telling you as you scroll: Do you feel connection and belonging, or comparison and longing?

Remember, as a woman your body's nature is connection, community, and cooperation. Josephine said, "This topic and conversation are the missing piece! We need daily mentoring for women and a strong sense of community." Now is the time to embrace the way you and your body have always wanted to live. How can you embody this in your relationships and serve as a role model for other women?

Share your newfound wisdom and connection with other women—start at home, then expand your influence. Become one of those women who refuses to engage in self-deprecation, body shame, or blame. Discuss this book in a book club or form an embodiment group or community where you can talk about your experiences and guide one another through the practices.

When you show up differently for your body, a ripple effect begins. Every change you make inspires a change in someone else. One thought, one word, one act of kindness or care for your body can spread to all bodies. This is how we begin to dismantle systems of harm and create systems of protection and care. As you heal, you're repairing and reprogramming years of intergenerational trauma by allowing your body to live differently in the world—the way the women in your lineage wished to live if they had the chance. We can do this together.

EMBODIED PRACTICE

We Belong Together

This meditation reminds you that you belong. You may engage in this practice seated or lying down. Place one hand on your heart and the other on your abdomen below your navel to connect with your center. Recite the following:

*As I awaken each day, may I acknowledge this breath, this sensa-
tion, this moment in my body. I am here, my body is here, we
are here.*
*As I go out into the world, may I acknowledge my body and
others' bodies through respect, compassion, and mystery.*
My body and your body have their own story to tell.
My body and your body carry their own pain and life experience.
*My body and your body are different, yet long for the same
belonging.*
*My body and your body are different, yet long for the same safety,
protection, and peace.*
May I move beyond my eyes so that I may see through my heart.
I see you, I feel you, I sense you.
I am here with you.

The Never-Ending Cycle

Even though you're nearing the end of this book, you're not at the end of your embodiment journey. Living embodied through body forgiveness is a never-ending cycle. Embodiment through body forgiveness is an ongoing journey that never truly reaches completion. It's an integral part of life. We are born embodied and our greatest wish is to remain so. This desire inspired me to write this book—not just to remind myself but to support the countless women who long for reconnection with their bodies.

As I wrote this final chapter I felt a blockage in my mind and a pit in my stomach. It's hard to conclude something I've worked on for so long. After four years of research and writing, ending it feels like saying goodbye to a close friend. My mind wants closure, but my body knows the truth.

The pit in my stomach comes from my body, which understands the difficult truths about this journey. I wish I could offer you a neat ending or a clear path to follow. But I can't, because such simplicity doesn't exist. I can't promise the world won't continue to distract, hurt, marginalize, or oppress you and your body. I can't guarantee your body won't change in size, ability, or health. I can't promise aging won't bring distress, sickness, or pain. I can't protect you from feeling let down, betrayed, or deceived by your body. There will be days when you lose hope and slip back into disconnection. There will be cycles of grief that require compassion and forgiveness—sometimes daily, sometimes moment to moment. Through all of this, something has shifted inside. Something has shifted between you and your body, even if it's just a glimmer of reconnection that reminds you your body is still here, waiting for you.

You gave your body a chance by picking up this book to learn and practice how to reconnect with your most compassionate and for-giving friend. What I can promise is that, even if it hasn't been easy, you and your body have come so far together. Something has grown and shifted. Your body lets you know you're on the right track with spontaneous messages of release and relief. Even if you wish the reconnection had happened earlier, your body doesn't care about such things—it only lives in the present moment, waiting for you, as it always will.

There will come a day when returning to your body feels easier and more natural, like coming home. Eventually you'll arrive home and choose to stay, recognizing it as a familiar and safe place—one that existed long before you were born. Here, you can rest and feel at ease. Here, you reconnect with your true self, and the busy mind fades into the background. Here, you can feel and express your body's true nature, vitality, and wisdom. Here, you feel protected, grounded, and strong, untouched by external forces. Here, your body speaks to you, and you can sense, feel, respond, and be guided by it. This is where you return to the essence of who you are, uniting with your body and spirit as one. All you need to do now is lean in and listen.

A Compassionate Commitment to Your Body

I've been with you from the start. I've never left. I know you never meant to leave me. I know you never meant any harm to me, just as I never meant any harm to you.

I've been here all along, even when you were made to feel afraid or ashamed of me. I know you never meant any harm to me, just as I never meant any harm to you.

I speak to you when I am struggling, sick, or in need. Even if you forget to listen, ignore me, or withhold from me, I know you never meant any harm to me, just as I never meant any harm to you.

I'm here when you cry and grieve for me to be different from what you want me to be.

I'm also here and ready to welcome you home whenever you are ready to join me.

I am here with you until the end of our journey together.

We never meant to cause each other harm.

EPILOGUE

When I Die

JENNIFER C. MUELLER, SOCIOLOGIST
AND EMBODIED EXPLORER

When I die, I hope someone will say
She loved her body!
Though the world made it hard
In so many different ways.

When I die, I hope someone will say
She knew her body as a loving home.
She knew how it cared for her,
Unfailingly, until the very end.

When I die, I hope someone will say
She saw God in everything and everyone,
Though it took her some time.

When I die, I hope someone will say
The trees were her friends. And the ancestors. And the birds.
The loved, the unloved, the seemingly unlovable.
She made friends with them all.

When I die, I hope someone will say
She befriended joy and she befriended pain.
And she better understood
The seemingly safe in-between.

When I die, I hope someone will say
She tried and tried and tried.
But then, without trying,
She found she was enough.

When I die, I hope someone will say
She did and did and did.
And then, she did less,
And was a little more.

When I die, I hope someone will say
She cared and cared and cared.
And then, she folded herself
Into the caring.

When I die, I hope someone will say
Softly
Gently,
Simply,
"She was."

LIST OF EMBODIED REFLECTIONS AND PRACTICES

9. EMBRACING BODY EQUANIMITY

10. EMBRACING EMBODIMENT

APPENDIX

PLAYLIST

At the end of most self-help books, you will typically find a list of resources for further learning. However, instead of providing a resource list, I wanted to offer you something that continues to promote spontaneous movement, joy, and reconnection with your body. I hope this playlist accomplishes that. Please feel free to add to it as we work together to grow an embodiment community.

You may access the playlist by searching for the name in Spotify or by following the link provided on the audio recording page:

PLAYLIST NAME:
Your Body Never Meant You Any Harm
PLAYLIST AUTHOR: Ann

AUDIO RECORDING PAGE:
www.shambhala.com/body-forgiveness-practices

NOTES

INTRODUCTION

1 Gabor Maté, *When the Body Says No: Exploring the Stress-Disease Connection* (Vintage Canada, 2019).

CHAPTER 1. UNDERSTANDING DISEMBODIMENT AND BODIES IN THE WORLD

1 Thich Nhat Hanh, "Thich Nhat Hanh on How to Heal Your Inner Child," *Lion's Roar*, August 4, 2025, https://www.lionsroar.com/healing-the-child-within/.

2 Ragen Chastain, "Paradigm Entrenchment in the Weight-Centric Paradigm," *Ragen Chastain Newsletter*, August 10, 2024, https://weightandhealthcare.substack.com/.

3 Emily Munro, Gabriella Wells, Rigel Paciente, Nicole Wickens, Daniel Ta, Joelie Mandzufas, et al., "Diet Culture on TikTok: A Descriptive Content Analysis," *Public Health Nutrition* 27, no. 1 (2024): e169, https://doi.org/10.1017/S1368980024001381.

4 Christy Harrison, "What Is Diet Culture?" *Christy Harrison* (blog), August 10, 2018, https://christyharrison.com/blog/what-is-diet-culture. Also discussed in her book, *Anti-Diet: Reclaim Your Time, Money, Well-Being, and Happiness Through Intuitive Eating* (Little, Brown Spark, 2021).

5 Sabrina Strings, *Fearing the Black Body: The Racial Origins of Fat Phobia* (New York University Press, 2019), 6.

6 National Eating Disorders Association, "Weight Stigma—the Root of Eating Disorders," 2019, www.nationaleatingdisorders.org/weight-stigma-root-eating-disorders/.

7 Sonya Renee Taylor, *The Body Is Not an Apology: The Power of Radical Self Love*, 2nd ed. (Berrett Koehler, 2021), 57.

8 The World Economic Forum, in collaboration with the McKinsey Health Institute, *Blueprint to Close the Women's Health Gap: How to Improve Lives and Economies for All*, Insight Report, January 2025, https://reports.weforum.org/docs/WEF_Blueprint_to_Close_the_Women%E2%80%99s_Health_Gap_2025.pdf, notes that "women spend 25 percent more time in poor health than men."

9 Lisa Bowleg, "The Problem with the Phrase 'Women and Minorities': Intersectionality—an Important Theoretical Framework for Public Health," *American Journal of Public Health* 102, no. 7 (2012): 1267–73, https://doi.org/10.2105/AJPH.2012.300750.

10 Sandra Lee Bartky, "Foucault, Femininity, and the Modernization of Patriarchal Power," in *Feminist Perspectives on Eating Disorders*, ed. Patricia Fallon, Melanie A. Katzman, and Susan C. Wooley (Guilford Press, 1994), 129–30.

11 Rudolph M. Bell, *Holy Anorexia* (University of Chicago Press, 1985), 21.

12 Marcia Germaine Hutchinson, "Imagining Ourselves Whole: A Feminist Approach to Treating Body Image Disorders," in Fallon, Katzman, and Wooley, *Feminist Perspectives on Eating Disorders*, 154–55.

CHAPTER 2. UNDERSTANDING EMBODIMENT

1 Nikki Mirghafori, "Death Is a Part of Life," *Tricycle: The Buddhist Review*, October 14, 2023, https://www.nikkimirghafori.com/single-post/death-is-a-part-of-life -tricycle-magazine-october-14-2023.

2 Thich Nhat Hanh, "Thich Nhat Hanh on How to Heal Your Inner Child," *Lion's Roar*, August 4, 2025, https://www.lionsroar.com/healing-the-child-within/.

3 J. L. Fitzpatrick, Charlotte Willis, Alessandro Devigili, Amy Young, Michael Carroll, Helen R. Hunter, and Daniel R. Brison, "Chemical Signals from Eggs Facilitate Cryptic Female Choice in Humans," *Proceedings of the Royal Society B: Biological Sciences* 287, no. 1928 (2020): 20200805, https://doi.org/10.1098 /rspb.2020.0805.

4 Maurice Merleau-Ponty, *The Phenomenology of Perception*, trans. Colin Smith (Humanities Press, 1962), 96.

5 David Abram, *The Spell of the Sensuous: Perception and Language in a More-Than-Human World* (Pantheon Books, 1996), 45.

6 Merleau-Ponty, *The Phenomenology of Perception*, 96.

7 Niva Piran, *Journeys of Embodiment at the Intersection of Body and Culture: The Developmental Theory of Embodiment* (Academic Press, 2017), 12. Also see Dr. Piran's article "Embodied Possibilities and Disruptions: The Emergence of the Experience of Embodiment Construct from Qualitative Studies with Girls and Women," *Body Image* 18 (September 2016): 43–60, https://doi.org/10.1016 /j.bodyim.2016.04.007.

8 JoAnna Hardy, *Not Booked, Not Busy, Just Not Coming: Body Wisdom*, Insight Meditation Society, Black, Indigenous, and People of Color Retreat, June 21, 2022, audio recording, https://dharmaseed.org/talks/71209/.

CHAPTER 3. UNDERSTANDING YOUR SENSORY BODY

1 Kaira Jewel Lingo, Valerie Brown, and Marisela B Gomez, *Healing Our Way Home: Black Buddhist Teachings on Ancestors, Joy, and Liberation* (Parallax Press, 2024), quoted in "Finding the Juicy and Joyful in Celibacy," *Tricycle: The Buddhist Review*, April 11, 2024, https://tricycle.org/article/black-buddhist-teachers-celibacy.

2 Maurice Merleau-Ponty, *The Phenomenology of Perception*, trans. Colin Smith (Humanities Press, 1962).

3 Cynthia J. Price and Christine Hooven, "Interoceptive Awareness Skills for Emotion Regulation: Theory and Approach of Mindful Awareness in Body-Oriented Therapy (MABT)," *Frontiers in Psychology* 9, no. 798 (2018), https://doi .org/10.3389/fpsyg.2018.00798.

4 Tara Brach, "*The Sacred Pause*," October 3, 2018, audio recording, https:// tarabrach.libsyn.com/the-sacred-pause.

CHAPTER 4. UNDERSTANDING YOUR BODY'S INTERNAL STORY

1   Tara Brach, *Embodied Awareness—Pain and Living Fully—Part 3*, Insight Meditation Community of Washington, DC, 2013, audio recording, https://www.tarabrach.com/embodied-awareness-pain-living-fully-part-3/.

2   Bessel van der Kolk, *The Body Keeps the Score: Brain, Mind, and Body in the Healing of Trauma* (Penguin Books, 2015), 21.

3   Stephen W. Porges, *The Pocket Guide to the Polyvagal Theory: The Transformative Power of Feeling Safe* (W. W. Norton, 2017).

4   Deb Dana, *Anchored: How to Befriend Your Nervous System Using Polyvagal Theory* (Sounds True, 2021), 141.

5   Dana, *Anchored*, 141.

6   Lara Briden, *Hormone Repair Manual: Every Woman's Guide to Healthy Hormones After 40* (Lara Briden, 2021).

CHAPTER 5. EMBODYING COMPASSION

1   Reginald A. Ray, "Tapping into the Body for Radical Change and Transformation," *Tricycle: The Buddhist Review*, December 1, 2016, https://www.tricycle.org/article/somatic-meditation/.

2   Kristin Neff, *Self-Compassion: The Proven Power of Being Kind to Yourself* (William Morrow, 2011), part 2.

3   Social and Health Research Center, Inc., "Diet Culture: A Brief History," April 4, 2022, https://sahrc.org/2022/04/diet-culture-a-brief-history/.

4   Jon Kabat-Zinn, *Full Catastrophe Living: Using the Wisdom of Your Body and Mind to Face Stress, Pain, and Illness*, rev. ed. (Bantam Books, 2013), 25–26.

5   Deb Dana, *Anchored: How to Befriend Your Nervous System Using Polyvagal Theory* (Sounds True, 2021), 141.

CHAPTER 6. EMBODYING GRIEF

1   Paula Arai, "Where Fear and Love Meet," *Tricycle: The Buddhist Review*, August 22, 2023, https://www.tricycle.org/article/grief-zen-ritual/.

2   Kristin Neff, *Self-Compassion: The Proven Power of Being Kind to Yourself* (William Morrow, 2011), 47.

3   Sonya Renee Taylor, *The Body Is Not an Apology: The Power of Radical Self Love*, 2nd ed. (Berrett Koehler, 2021), 50.

4   Chris Germer, "Shame and the Wish to Be Loved," Center for Mindful Self-Compassion, January 30, 2019, https://centerformsc.org/blogs/blog/shame-and-the-wish-to-be-loved.

5   Gabor Maté, *When the Body Says No: Exploring the Stress-Disease Connection* (Vintage Canada, 2019), 8–11, 173–80.

6   Rose Hackman, *Emotional Labor: The Invisible Work Shaping Our Lives and How to Claim Our Power* (Flatiron Books, 2023).

7   Family Caregiver Alliance, *Women and Caregiving: Facts and Figures* (National Center on Caregiving, Family Caregiver Alliance, 2021).

8   Susannah C. Coaston, "Self-Care Through Self-Compassion: A Balm for Burnout," *Professional Counselor* 7, no. 3 (2017): 285–97.

CHAPTER 7. EMBODYING FORGIVENESS

1   Mark Coleman, "Why Are We So Hard on Ourselves," *Tricycle: The Buddhist Review*, January 23, 2022, https://tricycle.org/article/meditation-self-forgiveness/.
2   Fred Luskin, *Forgive for Good: A Proven Prescription for Health and Happiness* (HarperOne, 2003).
3   Jack Kornfield, "Letting Go," July 1, 2022, jackkornfield.com/letting-go/.
4   Kate Johnson, "Making Friends with Yourself," *Tricycle: The Buddhist Review*, October 16, 2022, https://www.tricycle.org/article/making-friends-with-yourself/.

CHAPTER 8. EMBRACING PRESENCE

1   Martin Aylward, "The Freedom of Embodied Presence," *Tricycle: The Buddhist Review*, https://www.tricycle.org/dailydharma/the-freedom-of-embodied-presence/.
2   Ellie Lisitsa, "Emotional Attunement," The Gottman Relationship Coach, June 25, 2024, https://www.gottman.com/blog/self-care-emotional-attunement/.
3   Susan Bordo, *Unbearable Weight: Feminism, Western Culture, and the Body* (University of California Press, 1993).
4   Niva Piran, *Journeys of Embodiment at the Intersection of Body and Culture: The Developmental Theory of Embodiment* (Academic Press, 2017), 130.
5   Helen Tworkov, "A Refuge That No One Can Touch," interview by James Shaheen, *Tricycle: The Buddhist Review*, May 14, 2024, https://www.tricycle.org/article/helen-tworkov-tricycle-talks.

CHAPTER 9. EMBRACING BODY EQUANIMITY

1   Kimberly Brown, "Loving-Kindness for Control Freaks," *Tricycle: The Buddhist Review* 19 October 19, 2023, https://www.tricycle.org/article/loving-kindness-control-freaks/.
2   Cynthia J. Price and Christine Hooven, "Interoceptive Awareness Skills for Emotion Regulation: Theory and Approach of Mindful Awareness in Body-Oriented Therapy (MABT)," *Frontiers in Psychology* 9 (2018), article no. 798, https://doi.org/10.3389/fpsyg.2018.00798.
3   ESPN News Services, "Elena Delle Donne Listens to Body, Announces Retirement," April 4, 2025, www.espn.com/wnba/story/_/id/44531899/elena-delle-donne-listens-body-announces-retirement.
4   Sogyal Rinpoche, *The Tibetan Book of Living and Dying*, rev. ed. (HarperOne, 2002), 20.

CHAPTER 10. EMBRACING EMBODIMENT

1   Lekey Leidecker, "Some Things Are Felt Through the Body," *Tricycle: The Buddhist Review*, September 4, 2023, https://www.tricycle.org/article/lekey-leidecker-body/.

BIBLIOGRAPHY

Arai, Paula. "Where Fear and Love Meet." *Tricycle: The Buddhist Review*, August 22, 2023. https://www.tricycle.org/article/grief-zen-ritual/. Accessed 28 June 2025.

Aylward, Martin. "The Freedom of Embodied Presence." *Tricycle: The Buddhist Review*, [date unknown]. https://www.tricycle.org/dailydharma/the-freedom-of-embodied-presence/.

Bartky, Sandra Lee. "Foucault, Femininity, and the Modernization of Patriarchal Power." In *Feminist Perspectives on Eating Disorders*, edited by Patricia Fallon, Melanie A. Katzman, and Susan C. Wooley. Guilford Press, 1994.

Bell, Rudolph M. *Holy Anorexia*. University of Chicago Press, 1985.

Bowleg, Lisa. "The Problem with the Phrase 'Women and Minorities': Intersectionality—an Important Theoretical Framework for Public Health." *American Journal of Public Health* 102, no. 7, (2012): 1267–73. https://doi. org/10.2105/AJPH.2012.300750.

Brach, Tara, host, *Tara Brach*, podcast, "The Sacred Pause," December 29, 2023. https://www.tarabrach.libsyn.com/the-sacred-pause.

Brach, Tara. *"Finding True Refuge."* *Tricycle: The Buddhist Review*, Spring 2013. https://www.tricycle.org/magazine/finding-true-refuge/.

Brach, Tara. *"Embodied Awareness—Pain and Living Fully—Part 3,"* lecture given at Insight Meditation Community of Washington DC, 2013. https://www.tarabrach.com/pain-living-fully/. Audio recording.

Bradford, Billie, and Robyn Maude. "Fetal Response to Maternal Hunger and Satiation: Novel Findings from a Qualitative Descriptive Study of Maternal Perception of Fetal Movements." *BMC Pregnancy and Childbirth* 14, no. 288 (2014).

Briden, Lara. *Hormone Repair Manual: Every Woman's Guide to Healthy Hormones After 40*. Lara Briden, 2021.

Brown, Adrian, Stuart W. Flint, and Rachel L. Batterham. "Pervasiveness, Impact, and Implications of Weight Stigma." *eClinicalMedicine* 47 (2022): 101408. https://doi.org/10.1016/j.eclinm.2022.101408.

Capra, Fritjof. *The Tao of Physics: An Exploration of the Parallels Between Modern Physics and Eastern Mysticism.* 4th ed. Shambhala Publications, 2010.

Chah, Ajahn. *"Loving-Kindness for Control Freaks." Tricycle: The Buddhist Review,* [date unknown]. https://www.tricycle.org/dailydharma/letting -go-completely/.

Chastain, Ragen. "Paradigm Entrenchment in the Weight-Centric Paradigm." *Ragen Chastain Newsletter,* August 10, 2024.

Coleman, Mark. "'Learning to forgive takes time, sometimes years. So be patient as you weave a little forgiveness into your daily routine as a way of strengthening your capacity to forgive.'" *Tricycle: The Buddhist Review* (@tricyclemag), Twitter (now X), March 10, 2023. https://www.twitter .com/tricyclemag/status/1840074061822431638.

Cornaro, Luigi. *The Art of Living Long.* Translated by William F. Butler. Milwaukee, 1903. https://archive.org/details/artoflivinglongoocorniala /page/n1/mode/1up.

Dana, Deb. *Anchored: How to Befriend Your Nervous System Using Polyvagal Theory.* Sounds True, 2021.

"Elena Delle Donne Listens to Body, Announces Retirement." *ESPN News Services,* April 4, 2025. https://www.espn.com/wnba/story/_/id/44531899 /elena-delle-donne-listens-body-announces-retirement.

Farb, Norman, Jennifer Daubenmier, Cynthia J. Price, Tim Gard, Catherine Kerr, Barnaby D. Dunn, Anne Carolyn Klein, Martin P. Paulus, and Wolf E. Mehling. "Interoception, Contemplative Practice, and Health." *Frontiers in Psychology* 6 (2015). https://doi.org/10.3389/fpsyg.2015.00763.

Fisher, Norman. "Impermanence Is Buddha Nature." *Lion's Roar,* Aug 14, 2024. https://www.lionsroar.com/impermanence-is-buddha-nature/.

Fitzpatrick, John L., Charlotte Willis, Alessandro Devigili, Amy Young, Michael Carroll, Helen R. Hunter, and Daniel R. Brison. "Chemical Signals from Eggs Facilitate Cryptic Female Choice in Humans." *Proceedings of the Royal Society B: Biological Sciences* 287, no. 1928 (2020). https://doi .org/10.1098/rspb.2020.0805. PMID: 32517615; PMCID: PMC7341926.

Gershon, Livia. "When Dieting Was Only for Men." *JSTOR Daily*, January 2, 2017. https://daily.jstor.org/when-dieting-was-only-for-men/.

Hardy, JoAnna. *"Not Booked, Not Busy, Just Not Coming: Body Wisdom,"* recorded at *Black, Indigenous, and People of Color Retreat*, Insight Meditation Society Retreat Center, June 21, 2022. https://dharmaseed .org/talks/71209/.

Harrison, Christy. *Anti-Diet: Reclaim Your Time, Money, Well-Being, and Happiness Through Intuitive Eating*. Little, Brown Spark, 2021.

Hlava, Patty, John Elfers, Jeremy Bieber, Suruchi Maitra, Candy Burge, Andrea Howard, Rosario Carbajal, Mark Jamieson, and Amy Casey. "Reorienting Through the Body: The Correlation Among Self-Transcendent Emotion Experiences and Interoceptive Aware- ness." *Journal of Humanistic Psychology* (2024). https://doi.org/10.1177 /00221678241292482.

Hutchinson, Marcia Germaine. "Imagining Ourselves Whole: A Feminist Approach to Treating Body Image Disorders." In *Feminist Perspectives on Eating Disorders*, edited by Patricia Fallon, Melanie A. Katzman, and Susan C. Wooley. Guilford Press, 1994.

Johnson, Kate. "Making Friends with Yourself." *Tricycle: The Buddhist Review*, October 16, 2022. https://www.tricycle.org/article/making -friends-with-yourself/.

Kaas, Jon H. *"The Organization of Neocortex in Early Mammals."* In *Evolution of Nervous Systems*, edited by Georg F. Striedter, John Rubinstein, Jon H. Kaas, Leah A. Krubitzer, Theodore H. Bullock, and Todd M. Preuss. Elsevier Science, 2016.

King, Ynestra. "Healing the Wounds: Feminism, Ecology and the Nature/ Culture Dualism." In *Reweaving the World: The Emergence of Ecofeminism*, edited by Irene Diamond and Gloria Feman Orenstein. Sierra Club Books, 1990.

Kornfield, Jack. "Letting Go." *JackKornfield.com*, July 1, 2022. www.jackkornfield.com/letting-go/.

Lakoff, George. "Explaining Embodied Cognition Results." *Topics in Cognitive Science* 4, no. 4 (October 2012): 773–85. https://doi .org/10.1111/j.1756-8765.2012.01222.x.

Leidecker, Lekey. "Some Things Are Felt Through the Body." *Tricycle: The Buddhist Review*, September 4, 2023. https://www.tricycle.org/article/lekey-leidecker-body/.

Leitan, Nuwan, and Lucian Chaffey. "Embodied Cognition and Its Applications: A Brief Review." *Sensoria: A Journal of Mind, Brain and Culture* 10, no. 1 (July 2024): 1–7. https://doi.org/10.7790/sa.v10i1.384.

Lingo, Kaira Jewel, Valerie Brown, and Marisela B. Gomez. "Finding the Juicy and Joyful in Celibacy." *Tricycle: The Buddhist Review*, April 11, 2024. https://www.tricycle.org/article/black-buddhist-teachers-celibacy/.

Lisitsa, Ellie. "Emotional Attunement." The Gottman Institute, updated June 25, 2024. https://www.gottman.com/blog/self-care-emotional-attunement/.

Luskin, Fred. *Forgive for Good: A Proven Prescription for Health and Happiness*. HarperOne, 2003.

Maté, Gabor. *When the Body Says No: Exploring the Stress-Disease Connection*. Vintage Canada, 2019.

Matousek, Mark. "A Splinter of Love." *Tricycle: The Buddhist Review*, Fall 2003. https://www.tricycle.org/dailydharma/a-splinter-of-love/.

Mattingly, Jayne. *This Is Body Grief: Making Peace with the Loss That Comes with Living in a Body*. Penguin Life, 2025.

Mehta, Nandini. "Mind-Body Dualism: A Critique from a Health Perspective." *Mens Sana Monographs* 9, no. 1 (2011): 202–9. https://doi.org/10.4103/0973-1229.77436.

Merleau-Ponty, Maurice. *The Phenomenology of Perception*. Translated by Colin Smith. Humanities Press, 1962.

Mirin, Alison A. "Gender Disparity in the Funding of Diseases by the US National Institutes of Health." *Journal of Women's Health* 30, no. 7 (2021): 956–63. https://doi.org/10.1089/jwh.2020.8682.

Moccia, Lorenzo, Marianna Mazza, Marco Di Nicola, and Luigi Janiri. "The Experience of Pleasure: A Perspective Between Neuroscience and Psychoanalysis." *Frontiers in Human Neuroscience*, vol. 12 (2018). https://doi.org/10.3389/fnhum.2018.00359.

Neff, Kristin. *Fierce Self-Compassion: How Women Can Harness Kindness to Speak Up, Claim Their Power, and Thrive*. Harper Wave, 2021.

Neff, Kristin. *Self-Compassion: The Proven Power of Being Kind to Yourself.* William Morrow, 2011.

Oakes, Sean. "The Four Elements." *Spirit Rock*, published June 1, 2019. https://www.spiritrock.org/practice-guides/the-four-elements.

Pearl, Rebecca L. "Weight Bias and Stigma: Public Health Implications and Structural Solutions." *Social Issues and Policy Review* 12, no. 1 (2018): 146–82. https://doi.org/10.1111/sipr.12043.

Pike, Katharine M., and Peter E. Dunne. "The Rise of Eating Disorders in Asia: A Review." *Journal of Eating Disorders* 3, no. 33 (2015). https://doi.org/10.1186/s40337-015-0070-2.

Piran, Niva. "Embodied Possibilities and Disruptions: The Emergence of the Experience of Embodiment Construct from Qualitative Studies with Girls and Women." *Body Image* 18 (2016): 43–60. https://doi.org/10.1016/j.bodyim.2016.04.007.

Piran, Niva. *Journeys of Embodiment at the Intersection of Body and Culture: The Developmental Theory of Embodiment.* Academic Press, 2017.

Porges, Stephen W. *The Pocket Guide to the Polyvagal Theory: The Transformative Power of Feeling Safe.* W. W. Norton, 2017.

Price, Cynthia J., and Helen Y. Weng. "Facilitating Adaptive Emotion Processing and Somatic Reappraisal via Sustained Mindful Interoceptive Attention." *Frontiers in Psychology* 12, no. 578827 (2021), https://doi.org/10.3389/fpsyg.2021.578827.

Price, Cynthia J., and Christine Hooven. "Interoceptive Awareness Skills for Emotion Regulation: Theory and Approach of Mindful Awareness in Body-Oriented Therapy (MABT)." *Frontiers in Psychology* 9, no. 798 (2018). https://doi.org/10.3389/fpsyg.2018.00798.

Ray, Reginald A. "Tapping into the Body for Radical Change and Transformation." *Tricycle: The Buddhist Review*, published December 1, 2016. https://www.tricycle.org/article/somatic-meditation/. Accessed 28 June 2025.

Rowan, Timandra. "Diet Culture: A Brief History," *Social and Health Research Center, Inc.* April 4, 2022. https://sahrc.org/2022/04/diet-culture-a-brief-history/.

Shapiro, Lawrence, and Shannon Spaulding. "Embodied Cognition." In *The Stanford Encyclopedia of Philosophy*, edited by Edward N. Zalta and Uri Nodelman. Summer 2024 ed. Stanford University. https://plato.stanford.edu/archives/sum2024/entries/embodied-cognition/.

Simmons, Danielle. "Epigenetic Influences and Disease." *Nature Education* 1, no. 1 (2008): 6. https://www.nature.com/scitable/topicpage/epigenetic-influences-and-disease-895/.

Smith, Nicholas C. "Black-White Disparities in Women's Physical Health: The Role of Socioeconomic Status and Racism-Related Stressors." *Social Science Research* 99, no. 102593 (2021). https://doi.org/10.1016/j.ssresearch.2021.102593.

Sogyal Rinpoche. *The Tibetan Book of Living and Dying*. Revised and updated ed. HarperOne, 2002.

Strings, Sabrina. *Fearing the Black Body: The Racial Origins of Fat Phobia*. NYU Press, 2019.

Taylor, Sonya Renee. *The Body Is Not an Apology: The Power of Radical Self-Love*. 2nd ed. Berrett-Koehler, 2021.

Thich Nhat Hanh. "Thich Nhat Hanh on How to Heal Your Inner Child." *Lion's Roar*, August 4, 2025. https://www.lionsroar.com/healing-the-child-within/.

Tworkov, Helen. "A Refuge That No One Can Touch." *Daily Dharma, Tricycle: The Buddhist Review*, 14 May 2024. https://www. tricycle.org/dailydharma/a-refuge-of-your-own/. Accessed 28 June 2025.

Van der Kolk, Bessel. *The Body Keeps the Score: Brain, Mind, and Body in the Healing of Trauma*. Penguin Books, 2015.

Waheed, Nayyirah. *salt*. CreateSpace Independent Publishing Platform, 2013.

Whelan, Timothy. "'The Flesh and the Spirit': Anne Bradstreet and Seventeenth Century Dualism, Materialism, Vitalism and Reformed Theology." Georgia Southern University. *Unpublished manuscript*.

Wolfsdorf, David. *Pleasure in Ancient Greek Philosophy*. 1st ed. Cambridge University Press, 2013.

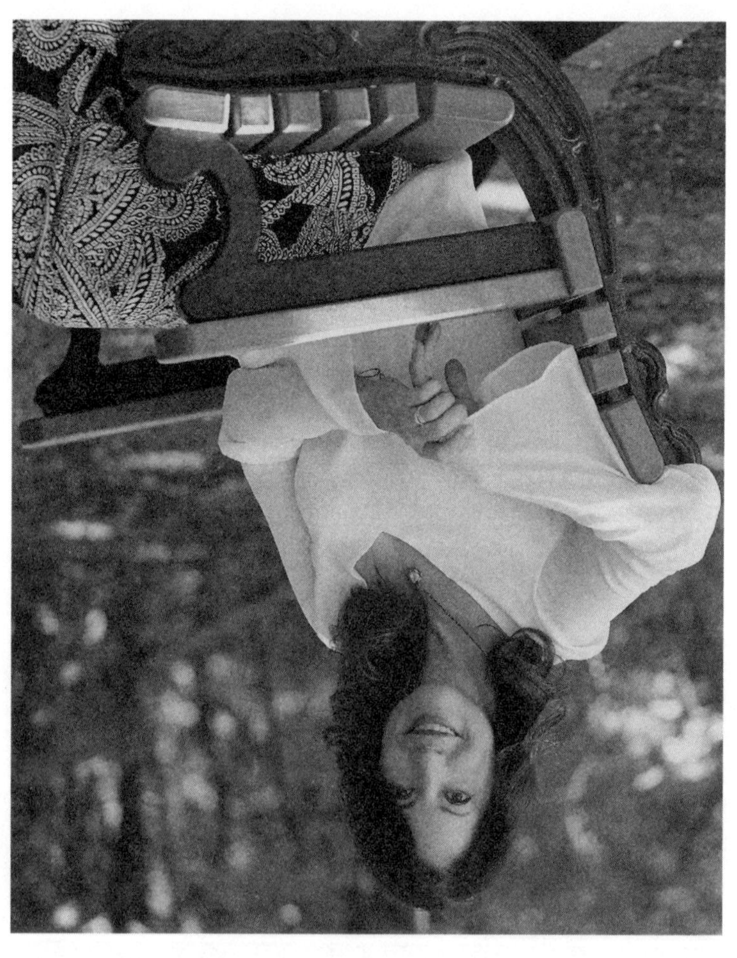

ABOUT THE AUTHOR

Ann Saffi Biasetti, PhD, LCSW, C-IAYT, is a transpersonal psychologist, licensed clinical social worker, and certified yoga therapist. She specializes in helping individuals heal their relationships with their bodies, food, and sense of self through somatic therapy, yoga therapy, and embodied self-compassion.

Ann is the creator of the Befriending Your Body Program, a somatic, self-compassion-based recovery program for disordered eating, and the author of *Befriending Your Body: A Self-Compassionate Approach to Freeing Yourself from Disordered Eating* and *The Awakening Self-Compassion Card Deck: 52 Practices for Self-Care, Healing, and Growth*. She contributed the chapter "The Process of Self-Compassion in Eating Disorder Recovery" to *Grounding Psychotherapy in Self-Compassion*.

Ann consults and lectures extensively on somatic psychotherapy, embodiment, polyvagal theory, and interoceptive awareness in the context of disordered eating and eating-disorder recovery. Additionally, she serves as an instructor with the Center for Mindful Body Awareness and the Self-Compassion in Psychotherapy (SCIP) Program. A featured Professional Education Systems Institute (PESI) presenter, she has appeared on multiple podcasts and trains professionals through the Befriending Your Body (BFYB) somatic certification training program.

Ann maintains a private therapy and consultation practice based in Saratoga Springs, New York, where she integrates mind-body modalities to facilitate holistic healing and personal growth. On any given day you can find her practicing and teaching yoga and meditation in her community and enjoying her family, friends, nature, animals, music, and embodied living.